donna hay

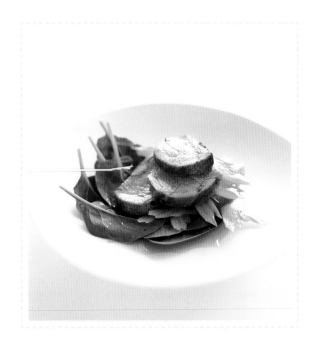

salads + vegetables

thank you

I have so many people to thank for helping with this book: Vanessa Pitsikas, for being a designer wise, composed and talented beyond her years; food editors Justine Poole, Steve Pearce and Jane Collings and their dedicated team of recipe testers for dishes that elicit oohs and aahs every time; copy editor Kirsty McKenzie for always asking the right questions; the amazing Con Poulos, talented Chris Court and all the other photographers whose images shine on every page; and, of course, to the *donna hay magazine* staff for being all-round superstars – your loyalty, creativity and professionalism help make donna hay a truly world-class brand. Many thanks must also be extended to Phil Barker and Peter Byrne at News Magazines; and to the team at HarperCollins. Thank you, thank you to friends old and new and my dear family. And to the men in my life: my wonderful sons Angus and Tom who make my heart soar, and my partner, Bill.

on the cover

front: roast tomato, chickpea and white bean salad, page 22
back: palm sugar salmon salad, page 32

Ecco

An imprint of HarperCollins*Publishers*

First American edition published 2008
First Australian edition published 2007
HarperCollins*Publishers*,
25 Ryde Road, Pymble, Sydney, NSW 2073, Australia
77-85 Fulham Palace Road, London W6 8JB, United Kingdom
2 Bloor Street East, 20th Floor, Toronto, Ontario M4W1A8, Canada
31 View Road, Glenfield, Auckland 10, New Zealand
10 East 53rd Street, New York, NY 10022, USA

Copyright © Donna Hay 2007. Design copyright © Donna Hay 2007
Photographs copyright © Con Poulos 2007 cover, pages 1, 4, 7, 9, 10, 11, 12, 13, 14, 15 (right), 16 (left), 17, 19, 20, 21, 23, 24, 25, 27, 29 (left), 30, 31, 33, 35, 37, 39 (left), 41, 42 (left), 43, 45, 47, 48 (right), 53 (right), 57 (left), 59, 61, 65, 66, 69, 71, 73, 74, 77, 79, 81, 83, 85 (left), 87, 96, back cover; copyright © Chris Court pages 15 (left), 16 (right), 38, 39 (right), 42 (right), 48 (left), 49, 51, 55, 56, 57 (right), 63, 75, 78 (right), 85 (right); copyright © Luke Burgess page 67; copyright © Hugh Stewart page 53 (left); copyright © Steve Brown page 60 (left); copyright © Brett Stevens page 29 (right); copyright © Kirsten Stecker page 60 (right); copyright © David Matheson page 78 (left).

Designer: Vanessa Pitsikas
Copy Editor: Kirsty McKenzie
Food Editors: Justine Poole, Steve Pearce, Jane Collings
Consulting Art Director: Sarah Kavanagh

Reproduction by Graphic Print Group, South Australia
Produced in Hong Kong by Phoenix Offset on 157gsm Chinese Matt Art.
Printed in China.

HarperCollins books may be purchased for educational, business, or sales promotional use. For information in the USA, please write: Special Markets Department, HarperCollins Publishers Inc., 10 East 53rd Street, New York, NY 10022.

Library of Congress Cataloging-in-Publication Data has been applied for.

ISBN-13: 978-0-06-156903-6

First Ecco Edition 2008
08 09 10 11 /IMP 10 9 8 7 6 5 4 3 2 1

donna hay

SIMPLE ESSENTIALS

salads + vegetables

ecco

An Imprint of HarperCollinsPublishers

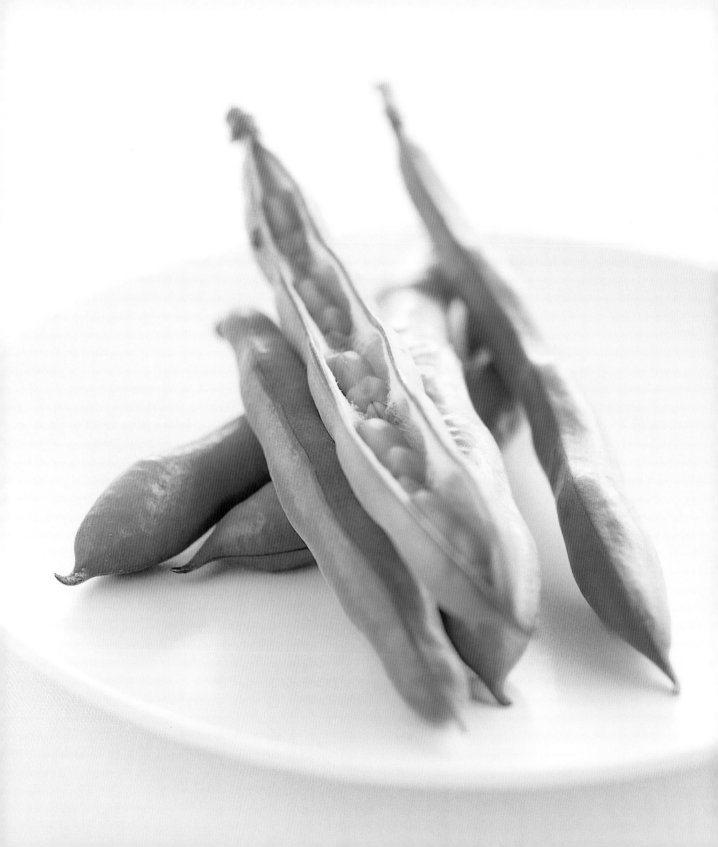

contents

introduction

In some parts of the world, the new season's potatoes are a Christmas treat to be dug up or bought from a roadside stall on Christmas Eve, gently scrubbed and served with due ceremony as the star of the festive feast. Tasting these potatoes, simply boiled and enhanced by nothing more than a sprinkling of sea salt and maybe a dob of butter, is to discover the humble spud in a whole new light. So it is with the entire vegetable kingdom. From asparagus to zucchini, if you use produce at its peak and treat it simply, even the staunchest meat lovers will regard it with renewed respect. We've created this book, so you too can kick-start conversions to the vegie lovers' cause. And there lots of options for meat lovers too, so I hope you enjoy cooking and sharing this selection.

Donna

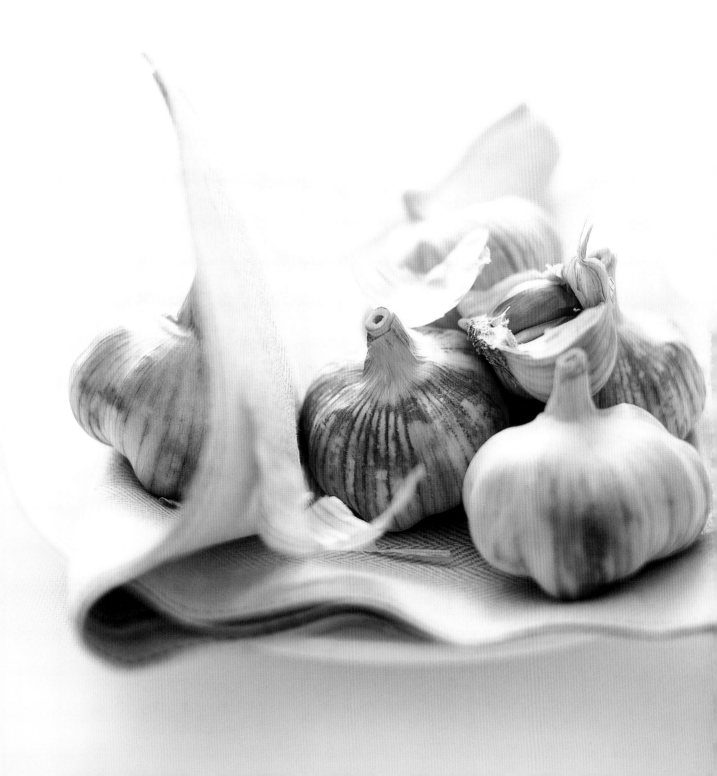

basics

When it comes to choosing salad leaves and vegetables, let "fresh is best" be your mantra. Trust your judgment and plan your menu around what looks best, because inevitably the vegies with the shiniest skin and most vibrant colour will taste the best. This section guides you through the most commonly used ingredients and provides expert tips on selection, storage and standby accompaniments.

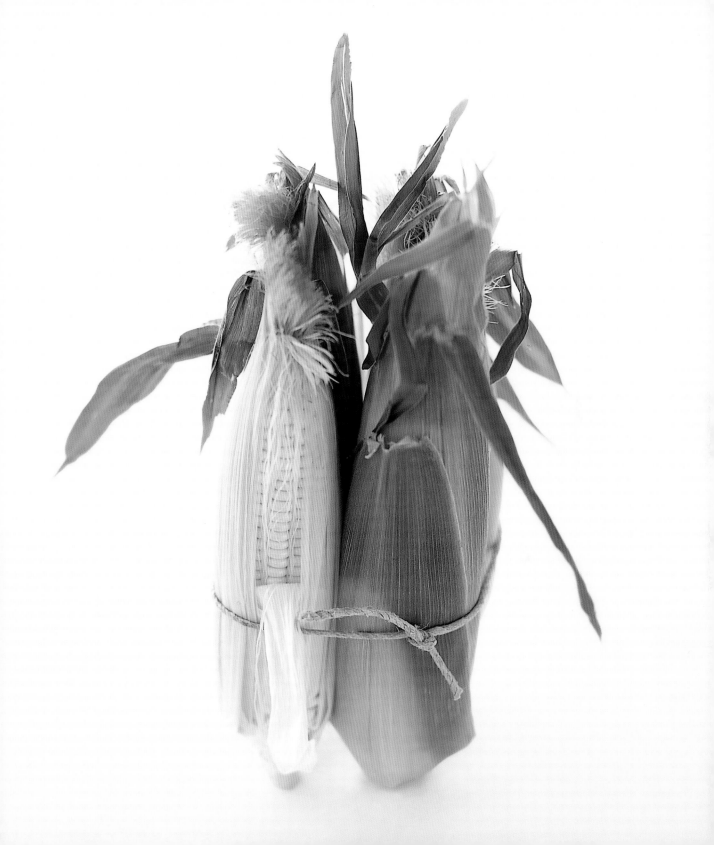

all about vegetables

Just picked may be best but most of us don't have the luxury of our own vegie patch. So cultivate your green grocer to make sure you always get the best produce at the peak of its season.

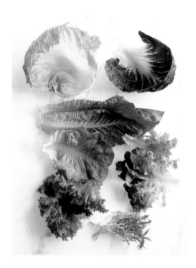

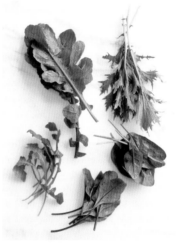

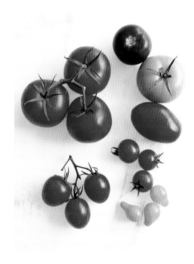

lettuces

The amazing array of lettuces means there is a lettuce for every season and reason. Some of the most popular varieties include (clockwise from top left) iceberg, radicchio, red and green oak leaf, frisée (curly endive), red and green coral, butter (mignonette) and cos (romaine). Freshly picked is best, but if you do have to store, seal whole lettuces in a plastic container before refrigerating. Wash and dry loose leaves before refrigerating in a vegetable storage bag. Discard any leaves which appear bruised or look slimy.

salad leaves

Salad leaves add flavour, colour and textural contrast to the mix. Popular options include (clockwise from top left) rocket (arugula/ruccola), mizuna, baby spinach, baby beet and wild rocket. Choose the freshest leaves available and balance peppery or bitter leaves with milder varieties. Reject any which are brown at the cut end or wilted in appearance. Wash and dry leaves before use. Store in the fridge in a vegetable storage bag or plastic bag lined with absorbent paper for up to two days.

tomatoes

Available year round, tomatoes peak in late summer and autumn. Popular types include (clockwise from top left) truss tomatoes, kumatos, green, roma, cherry, teardrop and baby roma tomatoes. When buying tomatoes, make sure they're heavy in the hand with blemish-free skins. Store at room temperature or place in the sun to finish ripening. Refrigeration will cause flavour loss. Truss fruit with the calyx intact can have better flavour because they are generally sold riper than other types and continue to ripen on the vine.

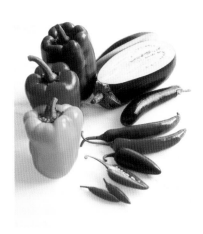

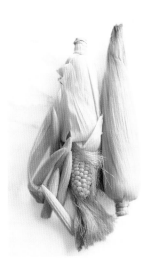

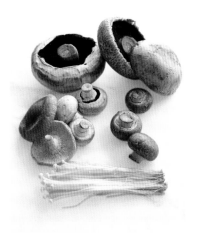

capsicums, chillies + eggplant

Among the delights of the warmer months are (clockwise from left) capsicums (bell peppers) in varying colours of ripeness from green to yellow and red, eggplants (aubergines), which come in regular oval shape or baby size, and chillies, including long green and red varieties as well as the more intense jalapeño and bird's eye. Shiny, wrinkle-free skin is an indicator of freshness and most can be kept in a vegetable storage bag in the fridge for several days.

corn

With little resemblance in flavour to its sweeter, larger counterpart, baby corn is largely used for its snappy texture and miniature appeal. It is the corn ear picked immature and very small so it's usually eaten whole. Buy corn on the cob and cook it as close as possible to when it's picked as it will be at its sweetest. Look for ears that are snug fitting and bright green with golden silk. The kernels should reach all the way to the tip and be plump and milky. Store corn protected by the husk and refrigerate for a few days at most.

mushrooms

Available year round but at their peak in autumn, mushrooms are an earthy delight that lend flavour and texture to soups, sauces, salads and stir-fries. Commonly encountered varieties include (clockwise from top left) flat (field) mushrooms, Portobellos, which are grown-up versions of Swiss browns, sculptural enokis (golden needles), shiitakes and buttons. Choose plump looking mushrooms that have no signs of bruising or sliminess. Storing in plastic makes them sweat and deteriorate, so store briefly in paper bags in the fridge.

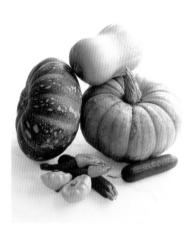

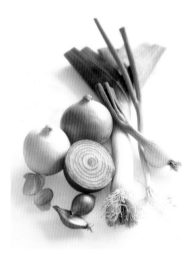

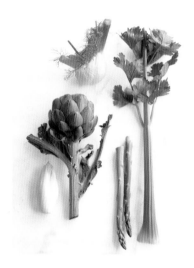

pumpkins + squash

This collection can be divided into winter squash, which need peeling, and summer squash, which don't. Winter squash include pumpkins such as (clockwise from left) the Japanese pumpkin, butternut and Queensland blue. Summer squash include Lebanese cucumbers, zucchini (courgette), zucchini flowers with the immature vegetable attached and green or yellow pattypan squash. Look for squash with glossy skins and store in the fridge for a few days only. Whole pumpkins keep well in an airy spot; refrigerate once cut.

bulbs

Onions can be grouped in two categories – dry onions that are allowed to mature in the soil before harvesting, and green onions, which are picked while still young. The dry set includes (on the left) white, brown and red (Spanish) onions, eschallots and their relative, garlic. Select firm, dry onions with no sprouts and store for several weeks in a cool, dry spot. Green onions (on the right) include the leek, thin green onion (scallion) and spring (salad) onions. Trim tops and roots and keep in the fridge for several days only.

shoot vegetables

As versatile as they are delicious, shoot vegetables are as at home in salads as they are in simmers and slow-cooked recipes. Favourites include (clockwise from top left) fennel, celery, asparagus, globe artichoke and witlof (sometimes called Belgian endive). Select the freshest examples you can find and avoid any that appear wilted, marked or bruised. Store in a vegetable storage bag in the crisper section of the refrigerator and use within a couple of days of purchase.

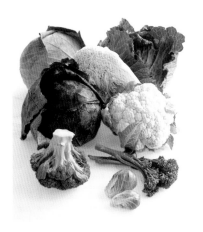

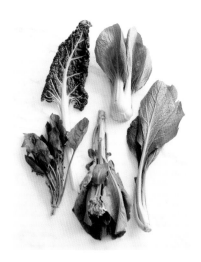

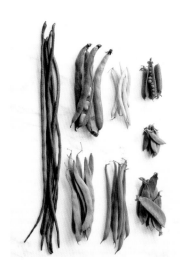

brassicas

The brassica family is available year round but comes into its own in winter, lending nutritious depth to hearty soups and slow braises. Alternatively, cook briefly to retain colour and flavour and serve as an accompaniment to roasts and grills or raw or lightly blanched in salads. Popular items include (clockwise from left) red, white, Savoy and Chinese cabbages, cauliflower, broccolini, Brussels sprouts and broccoli. Select brightly coloured vegetables with no sign of wilting and refrigerate for only a couple of days.

leafy greens

This collection lends variety and interest to our menus and its Asian members are now readily available. We love their versatility and speed of preparation – they can be poached, braised, steamed or added to soups and stir-fries. Popular varieties include (clockwise from top left) silver beet (Swiss chard), bok choy, choy sum, gai larn (Chinese broccoli) and English spinach. Choose bright green examples with crisp, rather than bendy, stems. Store in a vegetable storage bag in the crisper section of the refrigerator.

peas + beans

Among the more versatile goodies from the vegie patch, peas and beans are best picked young, served snapping fresh and simply prepared. They include (clockwise from left) snake beans, broad (fava) beans, yellow (butter) beans, peas in the pod, sugar snap peas, snow peas (mange tout), green and Roman beans. Select peas and beans that are bright in colour with no blemishes or signs of wilting. Store for no more than 2–3 days in a vegetable storage bag in the refrigerator and serve immediately after cooking.

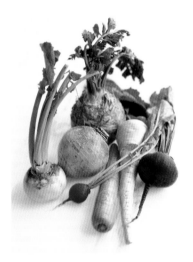

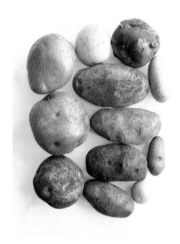

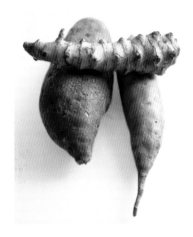

root vegetables

Although root vegetables are available year round, we tend to think of them as autumn and winter vegies because that's when we turn to them for use in soups, roasts and hearty, slow-cooked casseroles and stews. Popular roots include (clockwise from left) turnips, swedes, celeriac, beetroot, parsnip and carrot. The radish is more of a salad ingredient, lending peppery bite and colour contrast. Select firm vegetables with fresh-looking tops and store in a vegetable storage bag in the crisper section of the refrigerator.

potatoes

Although some are sold as all-purpose, broadly speaking, potatoes divide into two categories – waxy and floury. Waxy potatoes are low in starch and stay firm when boiled, so they are great for salads, serving whole or adding to casseroles. Floury potatoes are high in starch, so they're great for mashing, roasting and turning into chips. Consult your grocer or the packaging for the best variety for each recipe. Select firm potatoes with no marks, sprouts or green tinges and store in a dark, airy spot for up to several weeks.

tubers

From the popular orange-fleshed sweet potato, also known as kumara, to the more unusual white, yellow, red and purple varieties, sweet potatoes add distinctive sweetness to salads, roasts, mash, dips and pizza. They should be firm with no bruises on the skin. Keep for up to two weeks in a dark, well-ventilated spot. Knobbly Jerusalem artichokes are another tuber which can be roasted and mashed or used in soups. Store in the refrigerator for up to a week. After peeling, drop into accidulated water to stop discolouration.

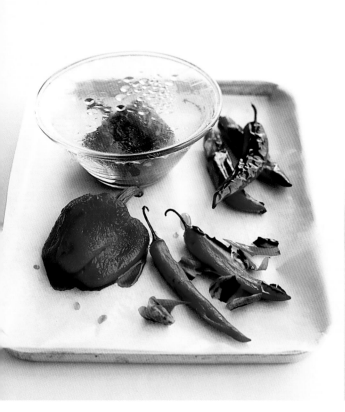

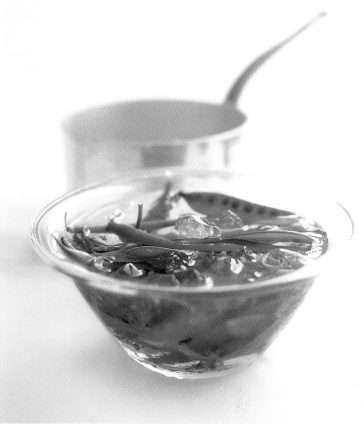

roasting capsicums and chillies

Roast capsicums (bell peppers) and chillies for a smoky flavour and rich colouring that makes a classic salad irresistible. Lay them out on a baking tray lined with non-stick baking paper, place in a preheated 200°C (400°F) oven until the skin starts to blacken, blister and move away from the flesh. Remove from the heat, place in a bowl and immediately cover with plastic wrap to make them sweat, so the skin peels off easily.

blanching greens

Preserve tenderness and crunch by briefly blanching spring vegetables. Peel, cut or trim away tough, woody stems, ends or skins and rinse the vegetables under cold water. Place them in a pot of rapidly boiling water and cook until they turn bright green or are just tender. Drain and serve immediately for hot vegies. For a side dish or salad, immerse the cooked vegetables in iced water to refresh the vegetables and stop the cooking process.

essential sides

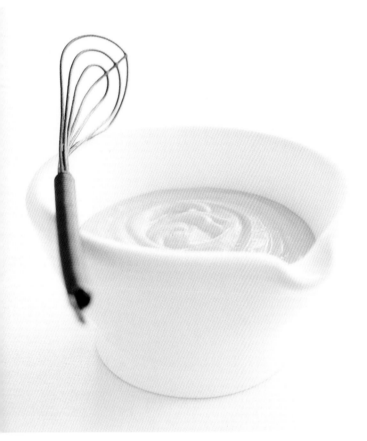

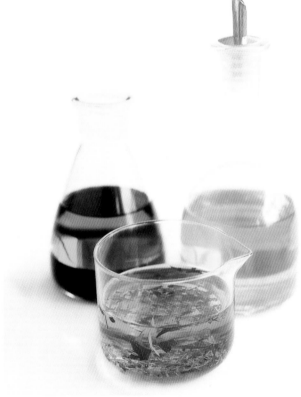

whole-egg mayonnaise + aioli

Process 1 egg, 1 tablespoon lemon juice, 2 teaspoons Dijon mustard, sea salt and ground white pepper in a food processor until combined. With the motor running, slowly pour in 1 cup (250ml/8 fl oz) oil and process until the mixture is thick. Makes 1¼ cups. For aioli, drizzle 1 head garlic with a little olive oil, wrap in foil and bake in a 180°C (350°F) oven for 30 minutes. Cool, squeeze garlic from cloves and fold through mayonnaise.

basic vinaigrette

Place ½ cup (125ml/4 fl oz) olive oil, 2 tablespoons white wine vinegar, sea salt and cracked black pepper in a bowl and whisk to combine. Vinaigrette is best freshly made, but will keep for 2–3 days in a sealed jar in the fridge. Bring back to room temperature and whisk to combine before using. Variations to the recipe include using red wine or balsamic vinegar and flavourings such as chopped herbs and seed or Dijon mustard.

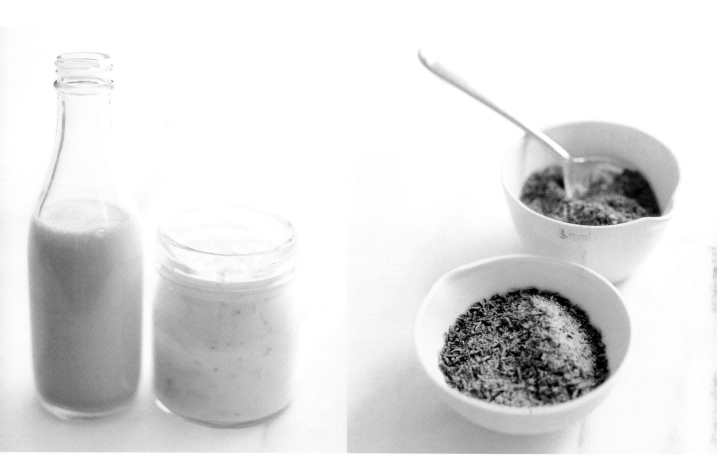

creamy dressings

Creamy dressings have a special affinity for crisp leaves and can elevate a simple salad to a supreme indulgence. The trick is to make sure the dressing has the consistency of single (or pouring) cream so it coats the leaves evenly rather than settling in dollops in the bowl. Add more liquid if it seems too thick. Recipes for the perennially popular buttermilk (or ranch) and caesar dressings are on page 88.

flavoured salts + rubs

To make fennel rosemary salt, combine 3 teaspoons fennel seeds, 3 teaspoons sea salt and 2 tablespoons rosemary in a small frying pan over medium heat. Cook for 1–2 minutes or until mixture is aromatic. Process in the bowl of a small food processor to crush. For cumin chilli salt, use 3 teaspoons cumin seeds, 3 teaspoons sea salt, 1 dried chilli and 1 teaspoon sweet paprika and prepare as above. Great on roasted vegetables.

salad starters + sides

It's hard to imagine a better asset for the cook than a snapping fresh salad. Simple to assemble, fast and easy to serve, salads can turn a snack into a meal or act as a light starter before a more substantial main. Toss with a lively dressing and you have an instant flavour boost or balance for a meal that has rich or fried components. From curtain raisers to support acts, we're sure this collection of recipes will become the stars in your repertoire.

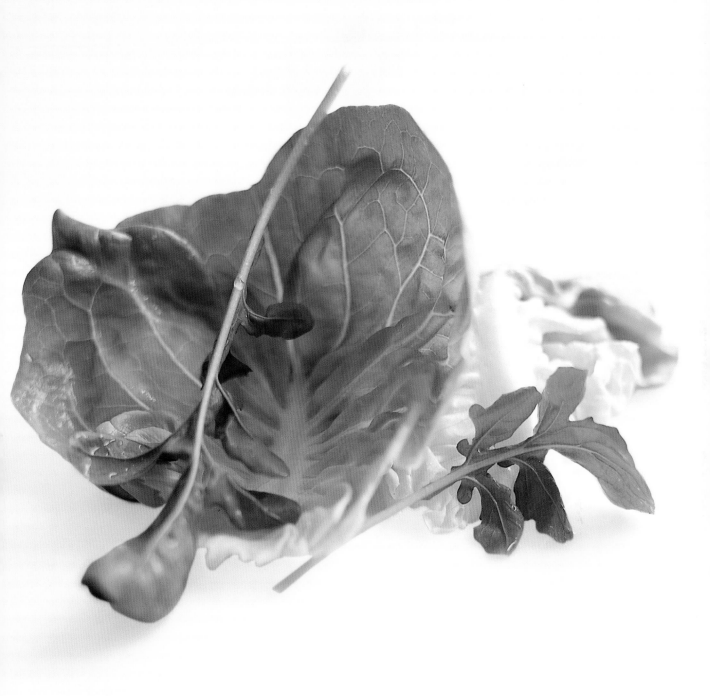

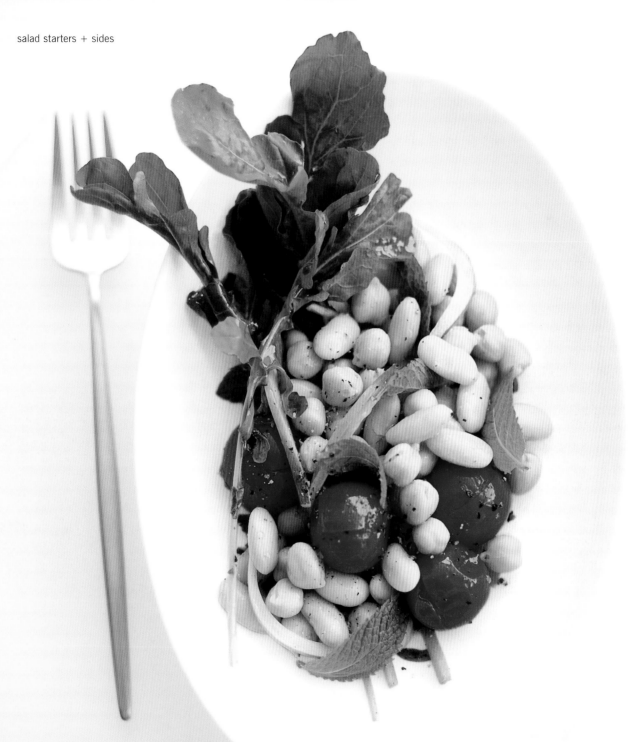

roast tomato, chickpea and white bean salad

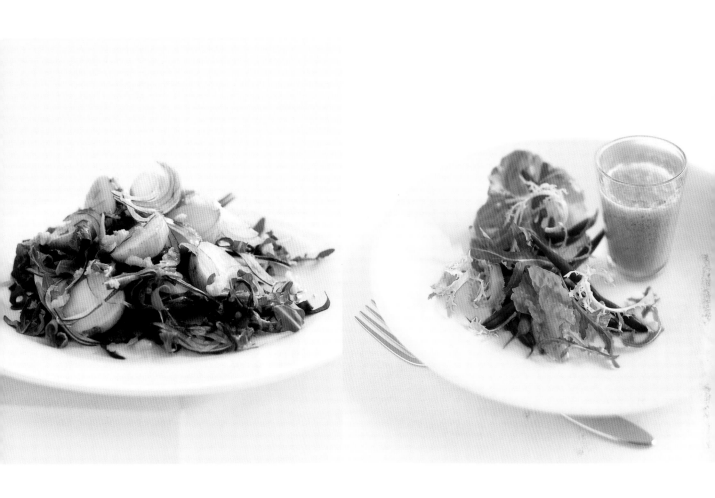

potato and wild rocket salad   French side salad

roast tomato, chickpea and white bean salad

250g (8 oz) cherry tomatoes
400g (14 oz) can chickpeas (garbanzos), rinsed and drained
400g (14 oz) can white beans, rinsed and drained
1 red onion, thinly sliced
2 cups mint leaves
70g (2½ oz) rocket (arugula) leaves
2 tablespoons lemon juice
2 tablespoons olive oil
sea salt and cracked black pepper

Preheat the oven to 200°C (400°F). Place the tomatoes on a baking tray lined with non-stick baking paper and cook for 5 minutes or until softened. Place the tomatoes, chickpeas, beans, onion, mint and rocket in a bowl and toss to combine. To serve, drizzle with the lemon juice and olive oil and sprinkle with salt and pepper. Serves 4.

potato and wild rocket salad

1kg (2 lb) baby/chat (new) potatoes, halved
100g (3½ oz) wild rocket (arugula) leaves, roughly chopped
½ red onion, finely sliced
1 teaspoon finely grated lemon rind
garlic dressing
4 cloves garlic, unpeeled
2 tablespoons olive oil
¼ cup (60ml/2 fl oz) white wine vinegar
¼ teaspoon sugar
sea salt and cracked black pepper

Preheat the oven to 180°C (350°F). To make the dressing, wrap the garlic in aluminium (aluminum) foil and bake for 35–40 minutes or until soft. Allow to cool, remove the skin and roughly chop the garlic. In a bowl, combine the garlic with the oil, vinegar, sugar, salt and pepper. Cook the potatoes in boiling water for 8 minutes or until tender. To serve, toss the potatoes with the rocket, onion, lemon rind and dressing. Serves 8.

French side salad

1 butter lettuce, outer leaves discarded, leaves separated
50g (1¾ oz) frisée (curly endive)
30g (1 oz) wild rocket (arugula) leaves
180g (6¼ oz) baby green beans, trimmed and blanched
French dressing
1½ tablespoons olive oil
1 tablespoon white wine vinegar
1 teaspoon Dijon mustard
sea salt and cracked black pepper

To make the French dressing, whisk the oil, vinegar, mustard, salt and pepper until combined. Toss the lettuce with the frisée, rocket and beans and place in bowls. Serve the dressing on the side. Serves 4.

red oak with bocconcini and prosciutto

8 slices crusty bread
1 clove garlic, halved
4 bocconcini, halved
2 red oak lettuces, outer leaves discarded, cut into wedges
8 slices prosciutto
balsamic vinegar, to serve
olive oil, to serve

Preheat a grill (broiler) to high. Toast the bread on both sides until crisp and golden. Rub with the cut garlic. Place the bocconcini on the lettuce wedges and wrap with a slice of prosciutto. Serve the lettuce wraps on the toast slices. Sprinkle with the vinegar and olive oil, if desired. Serves 4.

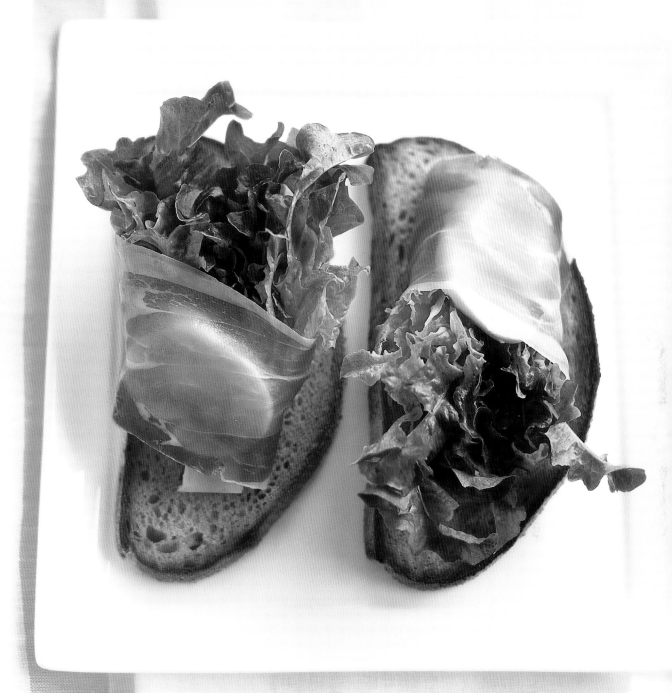

red oak with bocconcini and prosciutto

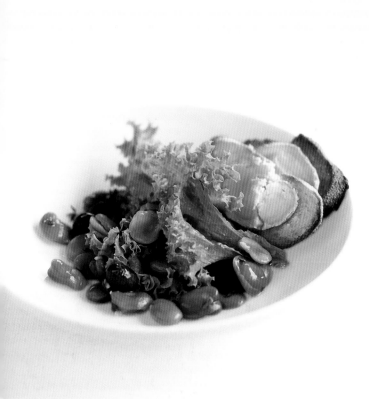

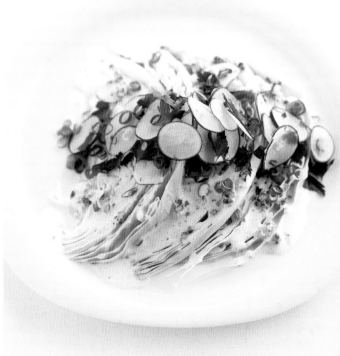

green coral salad with goat's cheese toasts

coleslaw

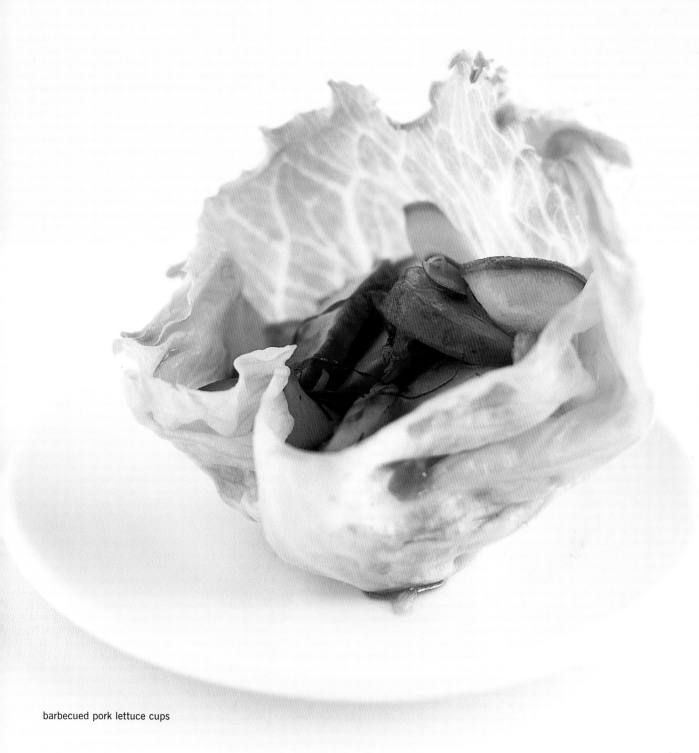

barbecued pork lettuce cups

green coral salad with goat's cheese toasts

8 thin slices sourdough baguette

40g (1½ oz) goat's cheese, cut into 8 rounds

1 green coral lettuce, outer leaves discarded, leaves separated

500g (1 lb) broad (fava) beans, blanched and skins removed

50g (1¾ oz) small black (Ligurian) olives

thyme dressing

1 tablespoon lemon juice

2 teaspoons thyme leaves

1 small clove garlic, crushed

1 tablespoon olive oil

sea salt and cracked black pepper

Preheat a grill (broiler) to high. Toast the baguette slices on both sides until crisp and golden. Top with the goat's cheese. Toss the lettuce with the broad beans and olives and divide among serving plates.

To make the dressing, whisk together the lemon juice, thyme, garlic, oil, salt and pepper. Pour the thyme dressing over the green coral salad and serve with the goat's cheese toasts. Serves 4.

coleslaw

¼ cabbage (375g/13¼ oz)

4 green onions (scallions), thinly sliced

¼ cup flat-leaf parsley leaves

8 radishes, thinly sliced

cracked black pepper

coleslaw dressing

1 egg

1 tablespoon white wine vinegar

2 teaspoons salted capers, rinsed

⅓ cup (80ml/2½ fl oz) vegetable oil

To make the dressing, process the egg, vinegar and capers in a food processor until combined. With the motor running, gradually pour in the vegetable oil until the dressing thickens slightly. Slice the cabbage into thin wedges and place on serving plates. Spoon over the dressing and top with the onions, parsley, radishes and pepper. Serves 4–6.

barbecued pork lettuce cups

¼ cup (60ml/2 fl oz) hoisin sauce

2 tablespoons soy sauce

¼ cup (60ml/2 fl oz) honey

1½ tablespoons Chinese rice wine

1 teaspoon Chinese five-spice powder

2 x 200g (7 oz) pork fillets, trimmed

2 Lebanese cucumbers, peeled into ribbons

2 tablespoons finely shredded mint leaves

1 long red chilli, seeded and finely sliced

4 iceberg lettuce leaves, trimmed into cups

hoisin dressing

1 tablespoon lime juice

1 tablespoon peanut oil

1 teaspoon brown sugar

1 teaspoon hoisin sauce

To make the dressing, whisk the lime juice, oil, sugar and hoisin in a small bowl until combined.

Combine the hoisin, soy, honey, rice wine and five-spice in a non-metallic bowl. Add the pork and mix to coat well. Cover and place in the fridge for 1 hour. Preheat the oven to 200°C (400°F). Drain the pork and place on a rack in a baking dish. Bake for 20 minutes or until cooked through. Slice. Place the cucumber, mint and chilli in a bowl and toss lightly. To serve, divide the salad between the lettuce cups, spoon over the dressing and top with the pork. Serves 4.

prosciutto and fennel salad

¼ cup (60ml/2 fl oz) lemon juice

⅓ cup (80ml/2½ fl oz) olive oil

sea salt and cracked black pepper

16 thin slices baguette, toasted

8 slices prosciutto

3 baby fennel, thinly sliced

shaved parmesan cheese, to serve

Combine the lemon juice, oil, salt and pepper in a jar or small bowl and set aside. To serve, layer the baguette, prosciutto, fennel and parmesan and spoon over dressing. Serves 4.

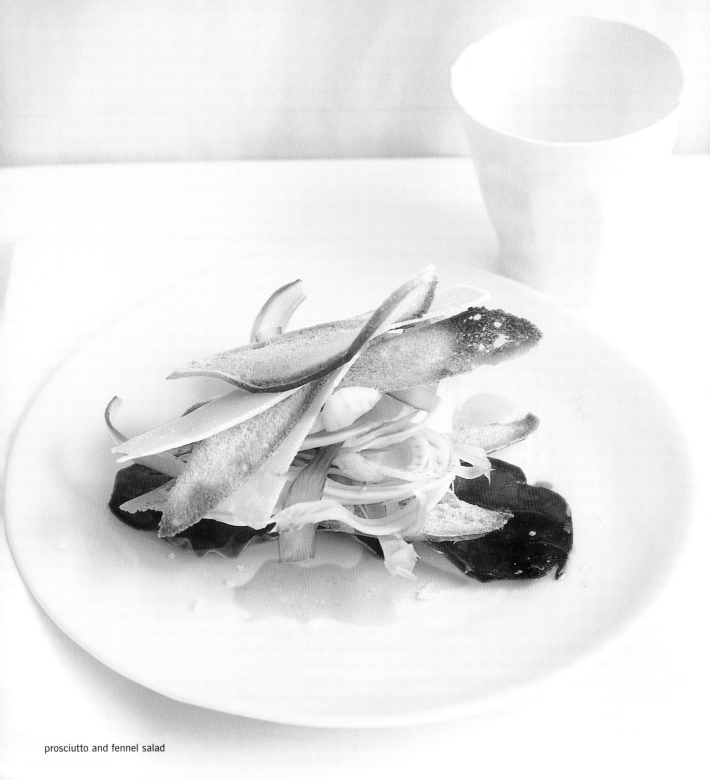

prosciutto and fennel salad

pan-fried haloumi and zucchini salad

1 tablespoon olive oil

20g (¾ oz) butter

1 clove garlic, crushed

2 yellow zucchini (courgette), thinly sliced

200g (7 oz) green beans, trimmed and blanched

250g (8 oz) haloumi cheese, sliced

lemon wedges, to serve

Heat the oil and butter in a medium non-stick frying pan over medium heat. Add the garlic, zucchini and beans and cook for 1–2 minutes or until tender and warmed through. Add the haloumi and cook for 1 minute each side or until golden. Serve the haloumi topped with the zucchini-bean mixture and with lemon wedges, if desired. Serves 4.

warm prawn and spring onion salad with wasabi dressing

2 tablespoons olive oil

20 medium green (raw) prawns (shrimp), peeled with tails intact

4 spring onions, trimmed and quartered lengthways

150g (5¼ oz) snow peas (mange tout), sliced

100g (3½ oz) enoki mushrooms, trimmed

sea salt and cracked black pepper

1 cup coriander (cilantro) sprigs

wasabi dressing

1 tablespoon wasabi paste

1 tablespoon white wine vinegar

¼ cup (60ml/2 fl oz) water

To make the wasabi dressing, place the wasabi, vinegar and water in a small bowl and whisk well to combine. Set aside.

Heat a large non-stick frying pan or wok over high heat. Add the oil and prawns and cook for 1 minute. Add the spring onions, snow peas, mushrooms, salt and pepper and cook for a further 2 minutes or until the spring onions are tender and the prawns are cooked through. Divide among bowls, spoon over the wasabi dressing and top with the coriander. Serves 4.

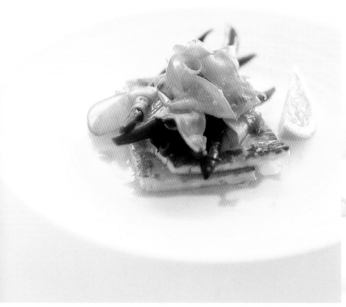

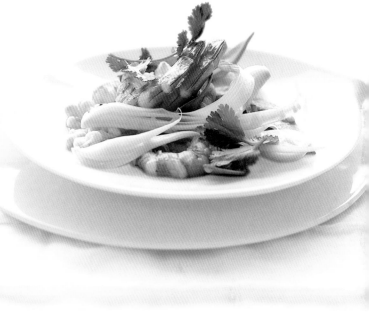

pan-fried haloumi and zucchini salad

warm prawn and spring onion salad with wasabi dressing

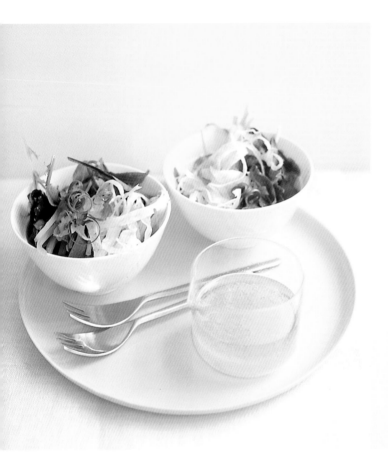

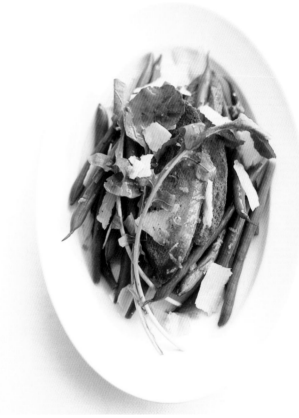

crispy fennel and celery salad

green bean, rocket and parmesan salad with crispy baguette

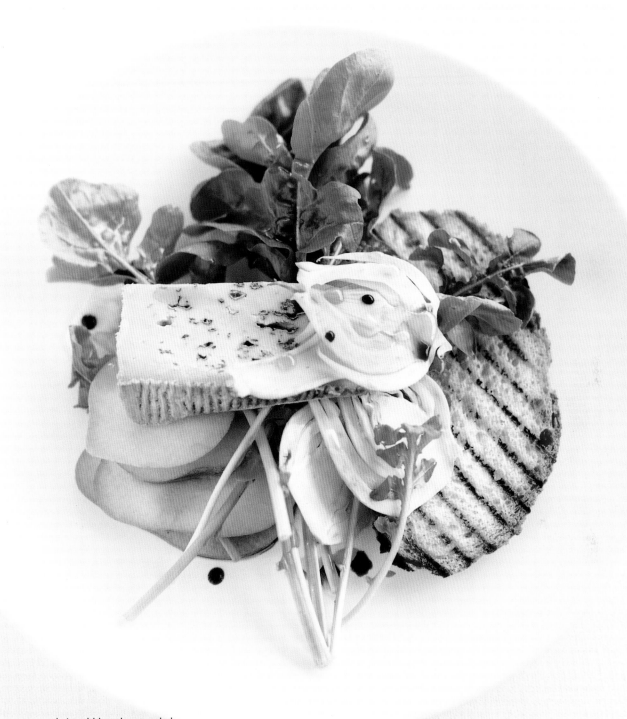

pear, rocket and blue cheese salad

crispy fennel and celery salad

1 fennel bulb, thinly sliced
½ cup chopped green onions (scallions)
3 stalks celery, thinly sliced
1 cup basil leaves, chopped
200g (7 oz) mixed baby salad leaves
lemon dressing
¼ cup (60ml/2 fl oz) lemon juice
¼ cup (60ml/2 fl oz) olive oil
1 teaspoon caster (superfine) sugar
sea salt and cracked black pepper

To make the lemon dressing, place the lemon juice, oil, sugar, salt and pepper in a small bowl and whisk to combine. Set aside. Place the fennel, green onion, celery, basil, mixed salad leaves in a bowl and serve with lemon dressing. Serves 6.

green bean, rocket and parmesan salad with crispy baguette

½ baguette, thinly sliced
olive oil, for brushing
250g (8 oz) green beans, trimmed and blanched
1 x 100g (3½ oz) bunch rocket (arugula), trimmed
40g (1½ oz) butter
1½ tablespoons lemon juice
1 teaspoon finely grated lemon rind
sea salt and cracked black pepper

Brush the baguette slices with olive oil and toast under a preheated hot grill (broiler) until golden. Layer the baguette on a serving platter with the beans and rocket. Combine the butter, lemon juice and rind, salt and pepper in a small saucepan over low heat and stir until the butter is melted. Spoon over the salad to serve. Serves 8.

pear, rocket and blue cheese salad

4 slices crusty Italian bread
150g (5¼ oz) rocket (arugula) leaves
2 baby fennel, thinly sliced
2 pears, thinly sliced
200g (7 oz) blue cheese, cut into wedges
balsamic vinegar, to serve
extra-virgin olive oil, to serve
sea salt and cracked black pepper

Grill or toast the bread until crisp. Arrange on plates with the rocket, fennel, pears and blue cheese. To serve, drizzle over a little vinegar and oil, and sprinkle with salt and pepper. Serves 4.

palm sugar salmon salad

2 tablespoons grated palm sugar
1 tablespoon finely grated lime rind
1 tablespoon lime juice
3 x 200g (7 oz) salmon steaks, skin removed
100g (3½ oz) watercress sprigs
200g (7 oz) sugar snap peas, blanched and halved
80g (2¾ oz) beansprouts
1 small red onion, sliced
1 long red chilli, seeded and thinly sliced
lime dressing
1½ tablespoons lime juice
1½ tablespoons palm sugar
1½ tablespoons fish sauce

Combine the palm sugar, lime rind and juice. Spoon over the salmon, coating well on both sides. Set aside for 5 minutes. Heat a medium non-stick frying pan over medium–high heat. Cook the salmon for 2 minutes on each side or until cooked to your liking. Flake the salmon into large pieces.

To make the lime dressing, mix together the lime juice, palm sugar and fish sauce in a small bowl.

Toss the watercress with the peas, beansprouts, onion and chilli. Gently combine with the flaked salmon and drizzle with the lime dressing. Serves 4.

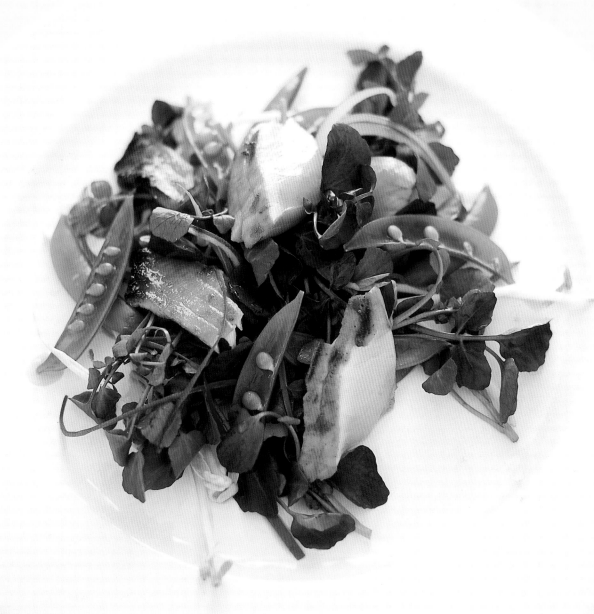

palm sugar salmon salad

Greek salad

4 vine-ripened tomatoes, quartered

2 Lebanese cucumbers, halved and sliced thickly lengthways

1 cup flat-leaf parsley leaves

¼ cup mint leaves, halved

1 cup kalamata or firm black olives

250g (8 oz) fetta cheese, sliced

cracked black pepper

red wine vinegar dressing

2 tablespoons olive oil

1 tablespoon red wine vinegar

sea salt and cracked black pepper

To make the red wine vinegar dressing, whisk together the oil, vinegar, salt and pepper in a small bowl.

Place the tomatoes, cucumbers, parsley, mint and olives in a serving bowl. Pour over the dressing and top with the fetta and cracked black pepper. Serves 4–6.

caesar salad

6 rashers bacon

1 cos (romaine) lettuce

1 quantity caesar salad dressing (recipe, page 88)

sea salt and cracked black pepper

¼ cup shaved parmesan cheese

croutons

¼ baguette, thinly sliced

olive oil, for brushing

1 clove garlic, halved

To make the croutons, preheat the oven to 180°C (350°F). Place the baguette slices on a baking tray, brush with the olive oil and bake for 10 minutes or until crisp and golden. Rub each slice with the cut garlic and set aside.

Place the bacon on a baking tray and cook under a hot grill (broiler) until crisp. When cooled, tear into large pieces. Trim the lettuce leaves, keeping the smaller inner leaves whole and roughly chopping the larger ones. To serve, toss together the lettuce, two-thirds of the dressing, the bacon, croutons, salt and pepper. Spoon over the remaining dressing and top with the shaved parmesan. Serves 4.

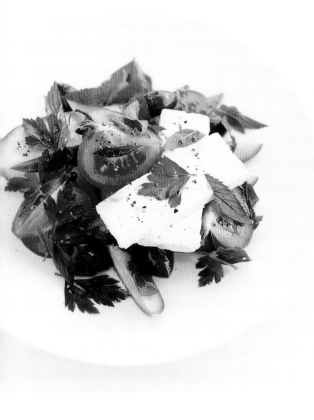

Greek salad

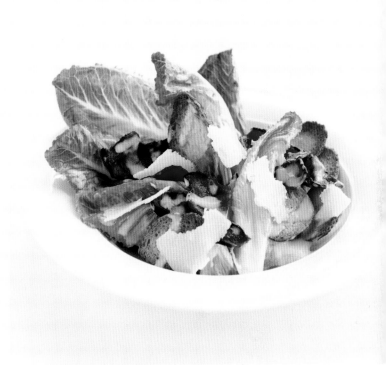

caesar salad

salad mains

For a healthy light lunch or main course during the warmer months, there is nothing easier to prepare or faster to serve than a salad. Take the market's freshest leaves and vegies, dress them up with meat or fish and accessorise with a sensational dressing for a meal that's guaranteed to draw enthusiastic responses every time. And, as the salads come together in one bowl or platter, reduced cleaning-up time is a welcome fringe benefit.

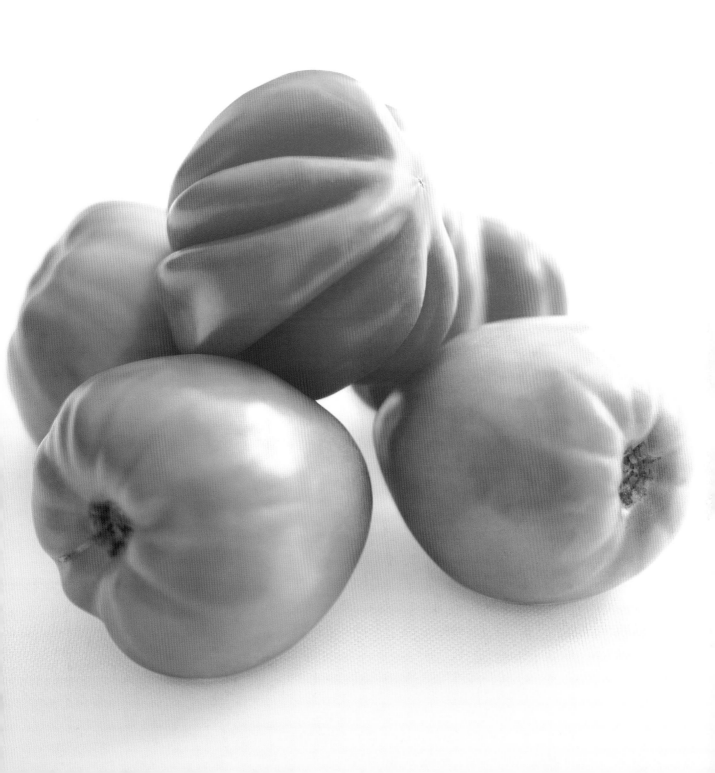

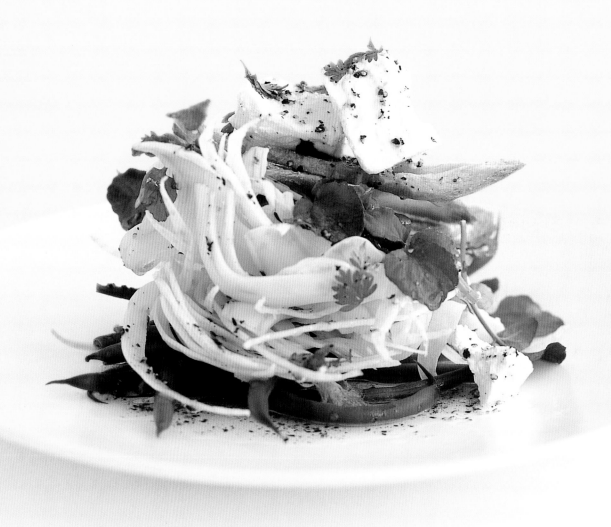

green bean, fennel and fetta salad

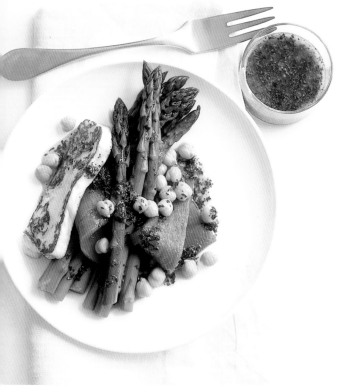

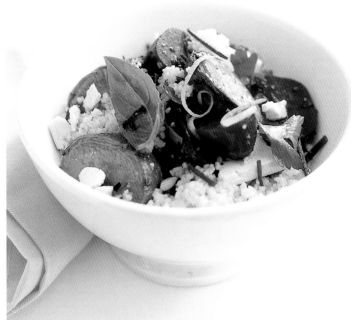

chervil and grilled haloumi warm salad

beetroot, fetta and sweet potato salad

green bean, fennel and fetta salad

200g (7 oz) green beans, blanched
1 x 300g (10½ oz) fennel, thinly sliced
70g (2½ oz) watercress
1 cup roughly chopped flat-leaf parsley leaves
6 thin slices sourdough bread, toasted
100g (3½ oz) fetta cheese, crumbled
2 tablespoons lemon juice
¼ cup (60ml/2 fl oz) olive oil
sea salt
½ teaspoon cracked black pepper

Layer the beans, fennel, watercress, parsley, sourdough and fetta on a serving plate. Combine the lemon juice, oil, salt and pepper in a small bowl or jar and drizzle over the salad. Serves 4.

chervil and grilled haloumi warm salad

2 tablespoons olive oil
8 spears asparagus, blanched
8 slices store-bought roast capsicum (bell pepper)
400g (14 oz) can chickpeas (garbanzos), drained and rinsed
250g (8 oz) haloumi cheese, sliced
chervil oil
2 cups chervil leaves
½ cup (125ml/4 fl oz) olive oil
1 clove garlic
sea salt and cracked black pepper

To make the chervil oil, place the chervil, oil, garlic, salt and pepper in a food processor and process until smooth. Set aside.

Heat a large non-stick frying pan over medium–high heat. Add half of the oil, the asparagus, capsicum and chickpeas and cook, stirring, for 2–3 minutes or until the asparagus and capsicum are warmed through. Remove from the pan and set aside. Place the remaining oil and the haloumi in the pan and cook for 1–2 minutes each side or until crispy and golden brown. Arrange the haloumi and asparagus mixture on plates and drizzle over the chervil oil to serve. Serves 4.

beetroot, fetta and sweet potato salad

300g (10½ oz) orange sweet potato (kumara), chopped
3 tablespoons olive oil
sea salt and cracked black pepper
850g (1 lb 14 oz) can whole baby beetroots, drained and halved
3 cups cooked couscous
150g (5¼ oz) fetta cheese, sliced
½ cup chopped chives
½ cup flat-leaf parsley leaves
¼ cup basil leaves
1 tablespoon lemon zest

Preheat the oven to 200°C (400°F). Combine the sweet potato, 1 tablespoon of the oil, salt and pepper in a bowl and toss to coat. Place on a baking tray and cook for 20–25 minutes or until cooked through and lightly browned. Allow to cool. Place the beetroot, couscous, fetta, chives, parsley, basil, lemon zest, sweet potato, remaining oil, salt and pepper in a bowl and gently toss to combine. To serve, divide the salad among the bowls. Serves 4.

Thai beef salad

650g (1 lb 7 oz) rump, fillet or sirloin steak, trimmed
oil, for brushing
150g (5¼ oz) salad leaves
2 x 100g (3½ oz) red onions, finely sliced
10 kaffir lime leaves, finely sliced
3 long red chillies, seeded and finely sliced
⅔ cup coriander (cilantro) leaves
⅔ cup mint leaves
⅔ cup basil leaves
1 quantity Thai dressing (recipe, page 91)
soy sauce, to serve

Brush the beef with a little oil and char-grill (broil), barbecue or pan-fry until cooked to your liking (medium rare is best for this salad). Set aside for 5 minutes, then slice thinly. Place the salad leaves, onions, lime leaves, chilli, coriander, mint and basil in a bowl and toss lightly. Toss the beef through the salad and pour over the dressing. Serve immediately with extra soy on the side, if desired. Serves 4.

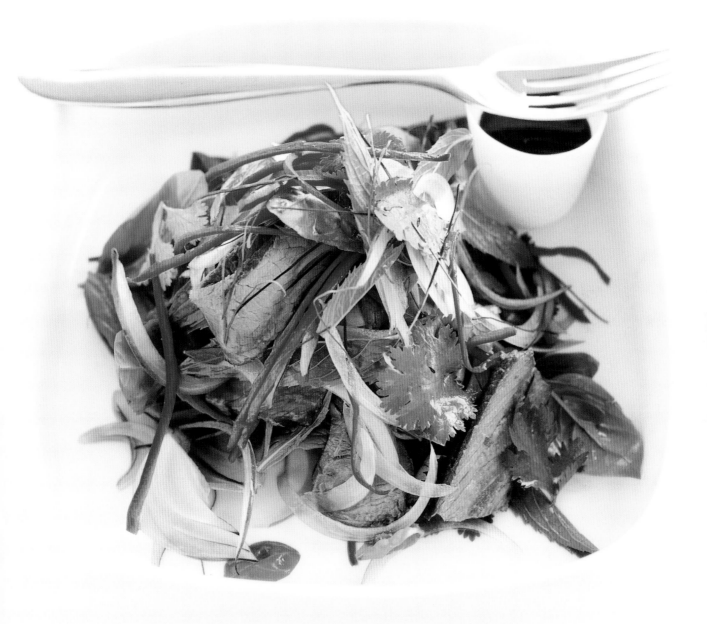

Thai beef salad

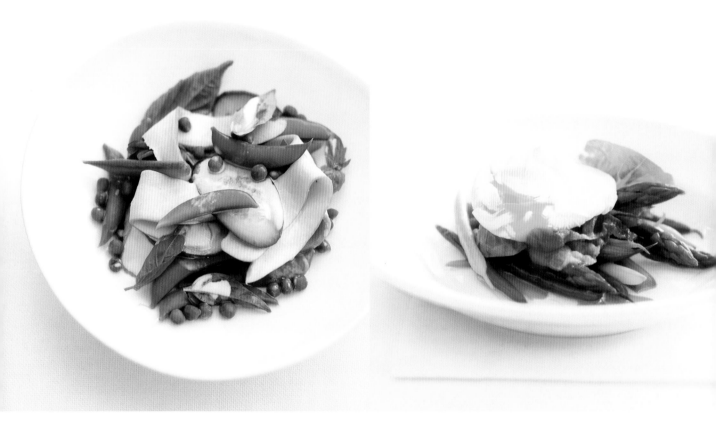

smoked chicken and pea salad with coconut dressing   asparagus, bean, bacon and egg salad

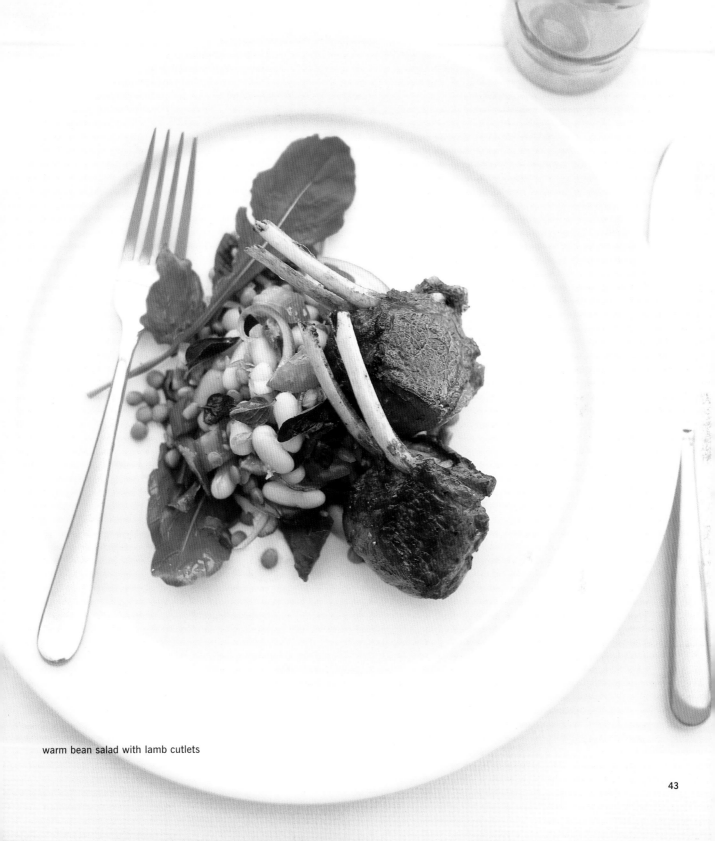

warm bean salad with lamb cutlets

smoked chicken and pea salad with coconut dressing

2 x 200g (7 oz) smoked chicken breast fillets, thinly sliced

100g (3½ oz) sugar snap peas, blanched

1 cup peas, blanched

1 cucumber, thinly sliced

1 cup basil leaves

coconut dressing

½ cup (125ml/4 fl oz) coconut cream

2 tablespoons lime juice

½ teaspoon fish sauce

1 teaspoon sugar

To make the coconut dressing, combine the coconut cream, lime juice, fish sauce and sugar in a bowl. Set aside. Place the chicken, sugar snap peas, peas, cucumber and basil in a bowl and toss to combine. To serve, divide among plates and spoon over the dressing. Serves 4.

asparagus, bean, bacon and egg salad

8 slices bacon, trimmed

150g (5¼ oz) yellow beans, trimmed

150g (5¼ oz) green beans, trimmed

12 spears asparagus, trimmed

1 tablespoon white wine vinegar

4 eggs

1 baby cos (romaine) lettuce, leaves separated

1 quantity white wine vinegar dressing (recipe, page 91)

Cook the bacon under a preheated hot grill (broiler) for 1–2 minutes or until crispy. Set aside. Blanch the yellow and green beans and the asparagus in a saucepan of salted simmering water for 1 minute or until just tender. Drain and refresh under cold running water, set aside. Heat a deep frying pan of water over low heat until just simmering. Add the vinegar and use a wooden spoon to create a gentle whirlpool. Crack each egg into a small bowl and gently slip into the water. Cook for 3–4 minutes, then remove the eggs with a slotted spoon. To serve, divide the bacon, beans, asparagus and lettuce among four plates and top each with a poached egg, then spoon over the dressing. Serves 4.

warm bean salad with lamb cutlets

8 double lamb cutlets, trimmed

3 tablespoons olive oil

2 cloves garlic, crushed

1 red onion thinly sliced

400g (14 oz) can white (cannellini) beans, rinsed and drained

400g (14 oz) can brown lentils, rinsed and drained

1 tablespoon red wine vinegar

½ cup oregano leaves

sea salt and cracked black pepper

1 x 100g (3½ oz) bunch rocket (arugula), trimmed

Brush the lamb with half the oil. Heat a large non-stick frying pan over medium heat. Cook the cutlets for 4–5 minutes each side or until cooked to your liking. Cover and set aside. Add the remaining oil, garlic and onion to the pan and cook for 1–2 minutes or until the onion is softened. Stir in the beans, lentils and vinegar and cook for 1 minute or until just warmed through. Stir through the oregano, salt and pepper and toss gently with the rocket. Divide the salad among four plates and top with the lamb. Serves 4.

pork, spinach and celery salad with orange dressing

2 tablespoons hoisin sauce

600g (1 lb 5 oz) pork fillet, trimmed

100g (3½ oz) baby spinach leaves

100g (3½ oz) celery, thinly sliced

orange dressing

¼ cup (60ml/2 fl oz) orange juice

¼ cup (60ml/2 fl oz) honey

1 tablespoon lemon juice

To make the orange dressing, combine the orange juice, honey and lemon juice. Set aside.

Heat a medium non-stick frying pan over medium–high heat. Brush the hoisin over the pork and cook for 3–4 minutes each side or until cooked through. To serve, slice the pork and arrange on the spinach and celery. Spoon over the dressing. Serves 4.

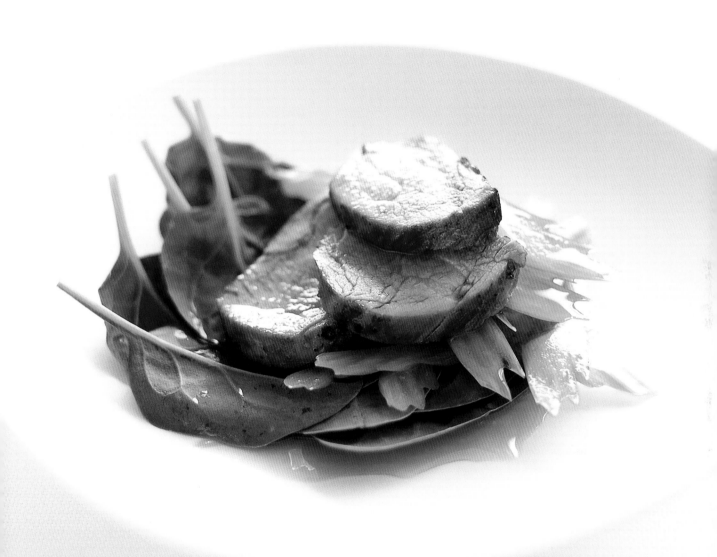

pork, spinach and celery salad with orange dressing

vegetable and crispy bread salad

8 slices wood-fired bread, roughly chopped

1 bunch chives, chopped

1 tablespoon finely grated lemon rind

70g (2½ oz) baby rocket (arugula)

200g (7 oz) marinated artichokes, drained and halved

200g (7 oz) black olives

200g (7 oz) semi-dried tomatoes, drained and chopped

200g (7 oz) roasted red capsicum (bell peppers), drained and sliced

2 tablespoons olive oil

2 tablespoons red wine vinegar

shaved parmesan, to serve

Preheat the oven to 200°C (400°F). Place the bread on a baking tray lined with non-stick baking paper and cook for 5 minutes or until golden and crispy. Place the bread, chives, lemon rind, rocket, artichokes, olives, tomatoes, capsicum, oil and vinegar in a serving bowl and toss to combine. Serve with shaved parmesan, if desired. Serves 4.

green olive and tomato couscous salad

1¼ cups (310ml/10 fl oz) chicken or vegetable stock

1 cup (180g/6¼ oz) couscous

20g (¾ oz) butter

800g (1¾ lb) vine-ripened tomatoes, chopped

100g (3½ oz) baby spinach leaves

¼ cup finely chopped mint

⅓ cup finely sliced green olives

150g (5¼ oz) fetta cheese, crumbled

balsamic dressing

2 tablespoons olive oil

1 tablespoon balsamic vinegar

sea salt and cracked black pepper

To make the balsamic dressing, combine the oil, vinegar, salt and pepper in a small jar or bowl.

To make the couscous, place the stock in a saucepan over medium heat and bring to a simmer. Place the couscous in a heatproof bowl and pour in the stock. Cover and set aside for 5 minutes before stirring with a fork to separate the grains. Stir the butter through the couscous. Toss the couscous with the tomatoes, baby spinach, mint, olives and fetta. Drizzle the dressing over the salad. Serves 4.

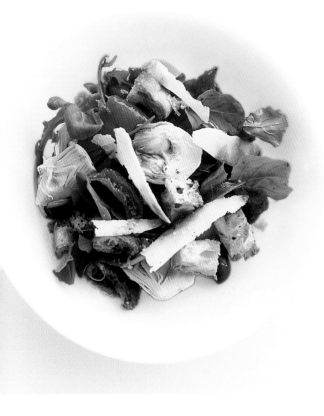

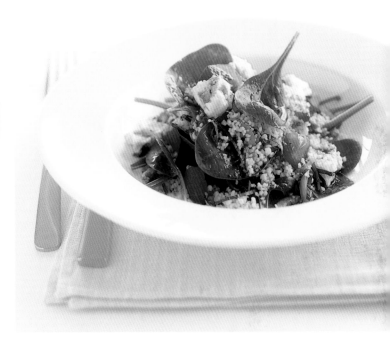

vegetable and crispy bread salad

green olive and tomato couscous salad

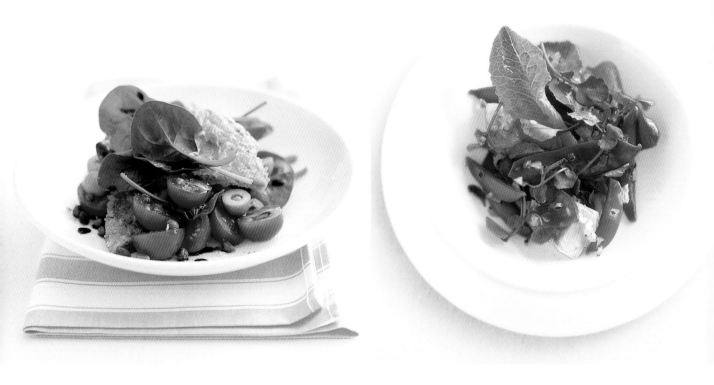

parmesan veal and spinach salad

pea, smoked salmon and watercress salad

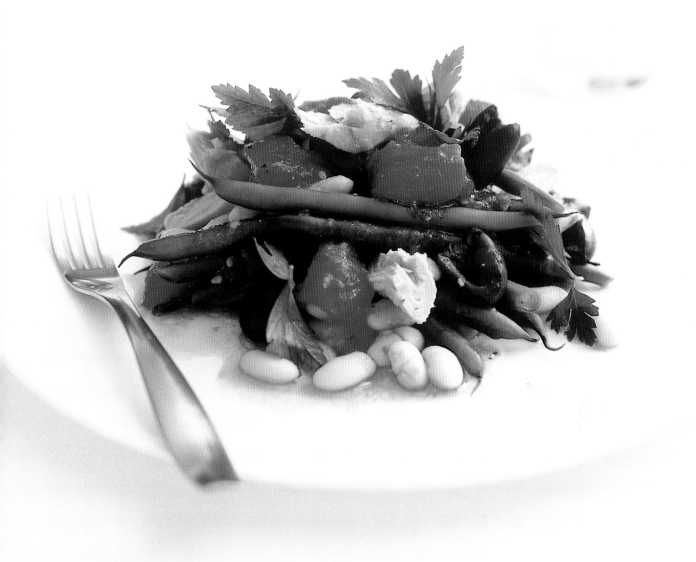

two bean and olive salad

parmesan veal and spinach salad

250g (8 oz) punnet cherry tomatoes, halved
⅓ cup green olives, pitted and halved
1 tablespoon salted capers, rinsed and drained
2 cups baby spinach leaves
1 tablespoon balsamic vinegar
2 tablespoons olive oil
⅓ cup (50g/1¾ oz) plain (all-purpose) flour
4 x 95g (3¼ oz) veal steaks
1 egg, lightly beaten
⅓ cup finely grated parmesan cheese

Place the tomatoes, olives, capers, spinach, vinegar and 1 tablespoon
of the oil in a bowl and toss to combine. Set aside. Place the flour on
a shallow tray. Dust the veal in the flour, dip into the egg and press into
the parmesan. Heat a large non-stick frying pan over high heat. Add
the remaining oil and cook the veal for 1 minute each side or until
cooked through and golden. Cut each veal steak in half and serve with
the spinach salad. Serves 4.

pea, smoked salmon and watercress salad

80g (2¾ oz) snow peas (mange tout), trimmed
100g (3½ oz) sugar snap peas, trimmed
1 cup watercress sprigs
1 tablespoon small mint leaves
1 baby cos (romaine) lettuce, leaves separated
4 x 100g (3½ oz) smoked salmon fillets, flaked
red onion dressing
30g (1 oz) butter
½ small red onion, finely chopped
2 teaspoons white wine vinegar

Cook the snow peas and sugar snap peas in boiling water for
2–3 minutes or until just tender. Drain, rinse under cold running
water and drain again. To make the dressing, stir the butter and
onion in a small saucepan over low heat until the butter is melted.
Stir the vinegar through. To serve, combine the snow peas, sugar snap
peas, watercress, mint and lettuce leaves and place in bowls. Top with
the salmon. Spoon over the dressing and serve immediately. Serves 4.

two bean and olive salad

1 cup roughly chopped flat-leaf parsley leaves
⅓ cup roughly chopped black olives
1 quantity roasted tomato sauce (recipe, page 88)
400g (14 oz) green beans, blanched
400g (14 oz) can white (cannellini) beans, rinsed and drained
185g (6½ oz) can tuna, drained

Place the parsley, olives, tomato sauce, green beans, white beans
and tuna in a bowl and gently toss to combine. Divide between plates
to serve. Serves 4.

lime and ginger salmon salad

2 tablespoons lime juice
1 teaspoon finely grated ginger
1 clove garlic, crushed
3 tablespoons olive oil
sea salt and cracked black pepper
4 x 200g (7 oz) salmon fillets
1 cup frozen broad (fava) beans, blanched with skins removed
1 cup frozen peas, blanched
2 green onions (scallions), thinly sliced
⅓ cup basil leaves
1 Lebanese cucumber, thinly sliced

Place the lime juice, ginger, garlic, oil, salt and pepper in a bowl and
whisk to combine. Place the salmon in a non-metallic bowl and pour
over half of the lime mixture. Marinate for 10 minutes. Combine the
beans, peas, green onions, basil and cucumber in a bowl. Heat a
non-stick frying pan over medium heat. Cook the salmon for 5 minutes
skin-side down. Turn and cook for a further 5 minutes. Break into
pieces and serve with the salad and the remaining lime mixture on
the side. Serves 4.

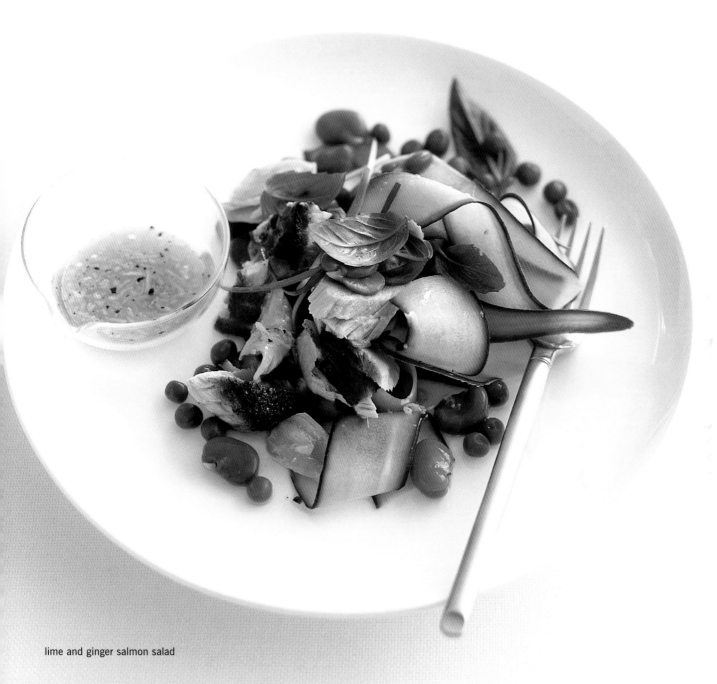

lime and ginger salmon salad

roast tomato, lemon and herb risoni salad

2 x 250g (8 oz) punnets teardrop tomatoes, halved
1 tablespoon olive oil
1 tablespoon finely grated lemon rind
500g (1 lb) risoni pasta
generous quantity shaved parmesan cheese, to serve
parsley and lemon dressing
1 cup flat-leaf parsley leaves, torn
1 cup mint leaves, torn
1 cup basil leaves, torn
2 green onions (scallions), finely sliced
2 tablespoons white wine vinegar
2 tablespoons lemon juice
½ cup (125ml/4 fl oz) olive oil
sea salt and cracked black pepper

Preheat the oven to 200°C (400°F). Place the tomatoes in a baking dish lined with non-stick baking paper. Sprinkle with the oil and lemon rind. Bake for 15 minutes or until soft. Cook the risoni in a saucepan of salted boiling water until al dente. Drain and rinse under cold running water until cooled.

To make the dressing, combine the parsley, mint, basil, green onions, vinegar, lemon juice, oil, salt and pepper. To serve, toss the dressing with the risoni. Top with the tomatoes and parmesan. Serves 6.

+ To make a more substantial meal, serve with grilled chicken or meat.

niçoise salad

12 baby/chat (new) potatoes, halved
300g (10½ oz) green beans, halved
400g (14 oz) tuna steaks
olive oil, for brushing
150g (5¼ oz) baby spinach or mixed salad leaves
2 tomatoes, cut into wedges
⅔ cup black olives
niçoise dressing
⅓ cup (80ml/2½ fl oz) olive oil
2 tablespoons red wine or sherry vinegar
2 teaspoons Dijon mustard
1 tablespoon chopped flat-leaf parsley
sea salt and cracked black pepper

To make the dressing, place the oil, vinegar, mustard, parsley, salt and pepper in a bowl and whisk to combine.

Place the potatoes in a saucepan of boiling water and cook for 5 minutes or until almost soft. Add the beans and cook for 2 minutes or until the beans and potatoes are tender. Drain and cool under running water. Brush the tuna with a little olive oil. Barbecue, char-grill (broil) or pan-fry for 1 minute each side or until the tuna is seared but not cooked all the way through. Set aside for 5 minutes then slice. Combine the potatoes, beans, leaves, tomatoes, olives and tuna on a serving plate and drizzle with the dressing. Serves 4.

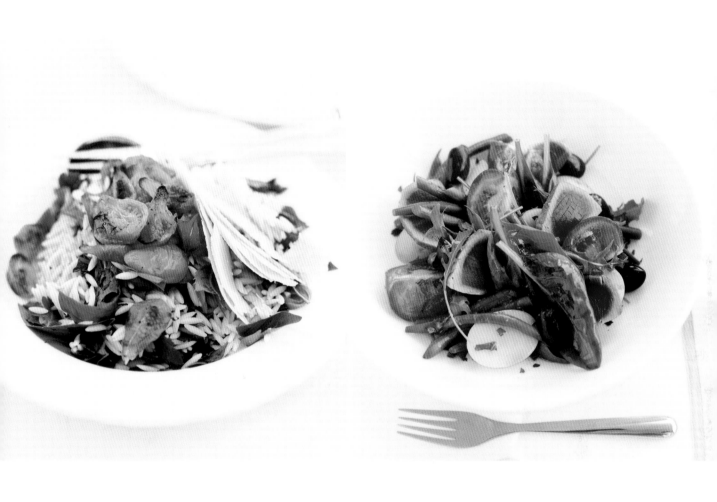

roast tomato, lemon and herb risoni salad

niçoise salad

vegetable starters + sides

Do your body and your taste buds a favour by increasing your vegie intake with this selection of our favourite vegie-based soups, starters and accompaniments. Starting with the freshest possible produce, we've given traditional treats a new-age update and more contemporary recipes a pared-back once-over to come up with a collection that is bound to have even fussy eaters clamouring for more.

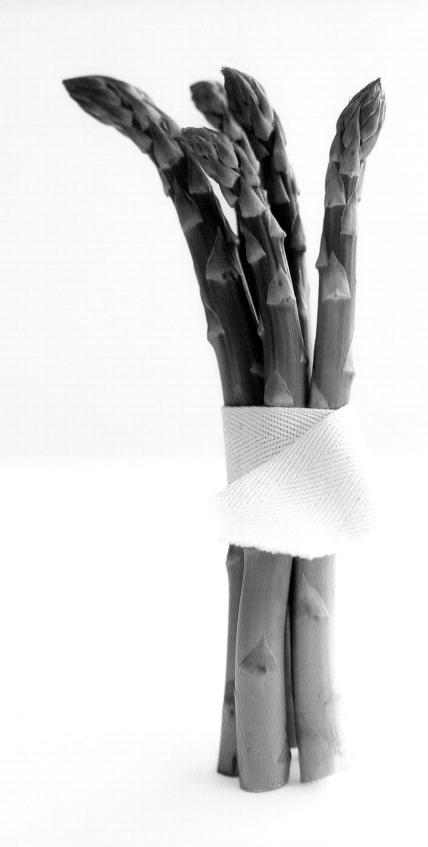

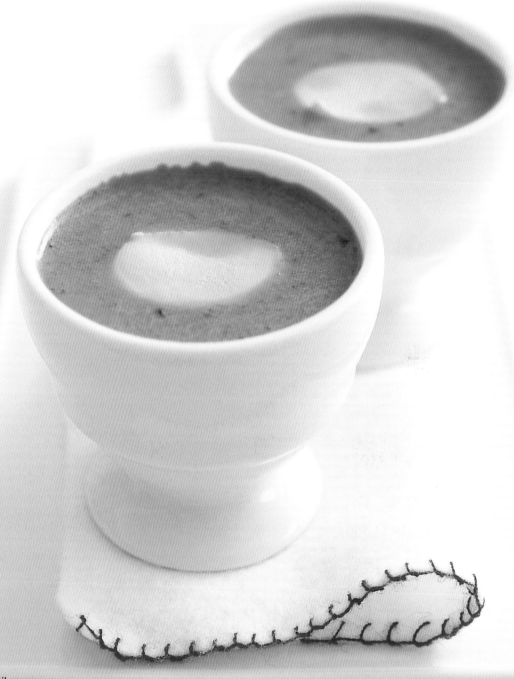

pea and basil soup

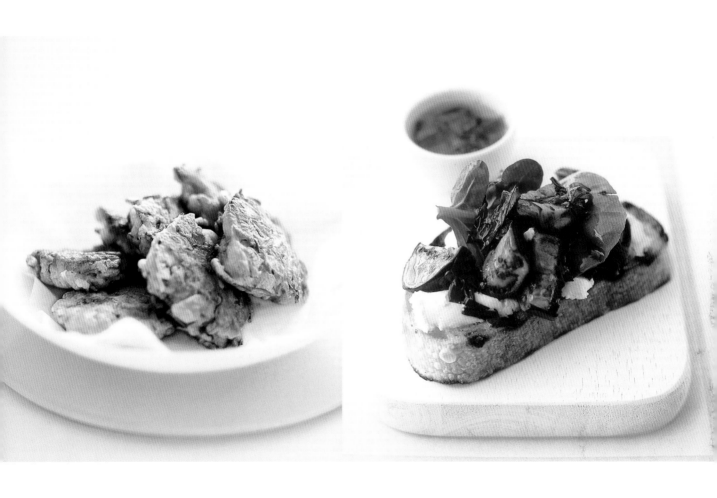

herb and spinach fritters   eggplant and basil bruschetta

pea and basil soup

40g (1½ oz) butter
1 brown onion, chopped
2 cups (500ml/16 fl oz) chicken or vegetable stock
2 cups frozen peas
sea salt and cracked black pepper
½ cup (125ml/4 fl oz) (single or pouring) cream
⅔ cup chopped basil leaves
2 bocconcini cheese, halved

Heat a medium saucepan over high heat. Add the butter and onion and cook for 3–4 minutes or until the onion is softened. Add the stock, peas, salt and pepper and bring to the boil. Reduce the heat to medium and simmer for 3–4 minutes or until the peas are tender. Stir through the cream and basil. Use a food processor or blender to blend the soup until smooth. Ladle the soup into bowls and top with the bocconcini. Serves 4.

herb and spinach fritters

1 cup (150g/5¼ oz) self-raising (self-rising) flour, sifted
2 eggs
20g (¾ oz) butter, melted
¼ cup (60ml/2 fl oz) milk
sea salt and cracked black pepper
¼ cup chopped chives
½ cup chopped basil leaves
½ cup chopped flat-leaf parsley leaves
1 cup baby spinach leaves
vegetable oil, for shallow-frying

Place the flour, eggs, butter, milk, salt and pepper in a large bowl and whisk to combine. Fold through the chives, basil, parsley and spinach. Place 2 tablespoons of the oil in a large frying pan over medium heat. Add tablespoons of the mixture to the pan and cook in batches for 1–2 minutes each side or until bubbles appear on the surface. Set aside and keep warm. Add another 2 tablespoons of the oil and repeat with the remaining mixture. Serves 4.

eggplant and basil bruschetta

12 slices sourdough bread
olive oil, for brushing
12 baby eggplants (aubergine), halved
½ cup basil leaves, chopped
⅓ cup flat-leaf parsley leaves, chopped
1 teaspoon salted capers, rinsed and drained
1 garlic clove, crushed
¼ cup (60ml/2 fl oz) red wine vinegar
2 tablespoons extra virgin olive oil
20g (¾ oz) rocket (arugula) leaves
150g (5¼ oz) goat's cheese

Brush the bread with the oil and cook on a preheated char-grill (broiler) for 2 minutes each side or until golden. Brush the eggplants with oil and char-grill (broil) for 5 minutes or until tender. Chop into pieces and set aside. Combine the basil, parsley, capers, garlic, vinegar and oil in a bowl. Combine the eggplant and rocket and toss with two thirds of the herb and garlic oil. Spread the goat's cheese over the bread and top with the eggplant mixture. Serve with the remaining herb and garlic oil. Makes 12.

butter-roasted cabbage

80g (2¾ oz) butter
1 eschallot, finely sliced
2 bay leaves
2 x 500g (1 lb) cabbages
¼ cup (60ml/2 fl oz) chicken or vegetable stock

Preheat the oven to 220°C (430°F). Melt the butter in a small saucepan over medium heat. Add the eschallot and bay leaves and cook until the eschallot is just tender. Cut the cabbages in half and place in a baking dish. Pour over the butter mixture and bake for 15 minutes. Reduce the temperature to 180°C (350°F). Pour over the stock and bake for 20 minutes. Serve with the pan juices. Serves 4.

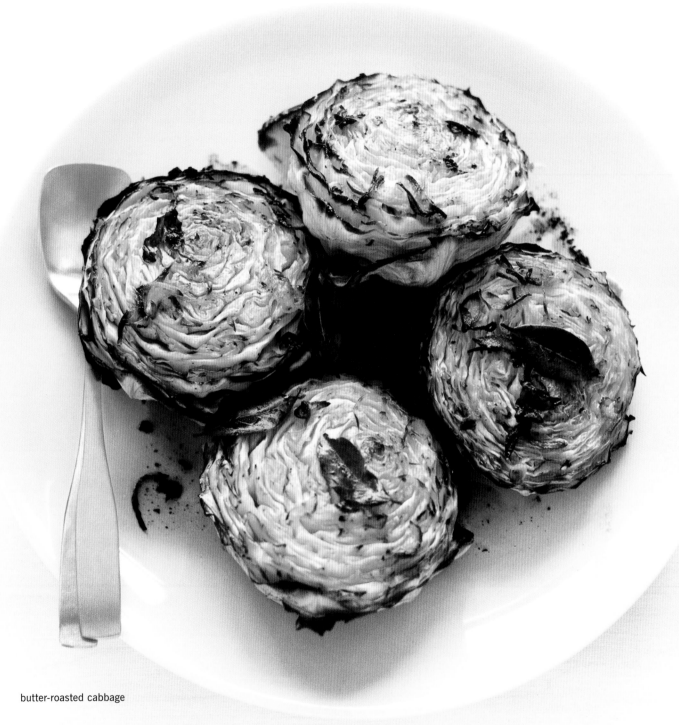

butter-roasted cabbage

spinach and ricotta triangles

100g (3½ oz) frozen spinach, defrosted
250g (8 oz) ricotta cheese
½ cup grated mozzarella cheese
2 teaspoons finely grated lemon rind
sea salt and cracked black pepper
6 pieces rectangular flat bread

Preheat the oven to 200°C (400°F). Drain the spinach well and place in a bowl with the ricotta, mozzarella, lemon rind, salt and pepper. Place ¼ cup of the spinach mixture on each piece of the bread and fold to enclose. Place on a baking tray lined with non-stick baking paper and bake for 10 minutes or until crisp and golden. Cut in half to form triangles. Serves 6.

silver beet, pea and pancetta soup

1 teaspoon vegetable oil
4 slices pancetta, chopped
1 small onion, chopped
2 cups (500ml/16 fl oz) chicken or vegetable stock
350g (12¼ oz) silver beet (swiss chard), trimmed and
   roughly chopped
2 cups frozen green peas
½ cup (125ml/4 fl oz) (single or pouring) cream
2 teaspoons lemon juice
cracked black pepper
soft goat's cheese, to serve

Place the oil, pancetta and onion in a saucepan over medium heat and cook for 3 minutes or until soft. Add the stock, increase the heat, cover and bring to the boil. Add the silver beet and peas and cook for 4 minutes or until tender. Stir through the cream, lemon juice and pepper. Blend in batches until smooth. To serve, pour into bowls and top with a slice of goat's cheese. Serves 2.

crunchy baby potatoes

24 baby/chat (new) potatoes
¼ cup (60ml/2 fl oz) olive oil
sea salt and cracked black pepper

Preheat the oven to 200°C (400°F). Use a small sharp knife to cut thin slices into the potato, ensuring you don't cut all the way through. Place the potatoes in a bowl with the oil, salt and pepper and toss to coat. Place in a baking dish and roast for 35–40 minutes or until golden and crunchy. Serves 6.

mushroom and sage butter bruschetta

6 slices sourdough bread
olive oil, for brushing
15g (½ oz) butter
1 teaspoon olive oil
6 field mushrooms
¼ cup sage leaves
1 garlic clove, thinly sliced
220g (7¾ oz) fresh buffalo mozzarella cheese, sliced

Brush the bread with olive oil and cook on a preheated grill (broiler) for 2 minutes each side or until golden. Heat a medium non-stick frying pan over high heat. Add the butter, oil and mushrooms and cook for 5 minutes or until the mushrooms are tender. Remove the mushrooms and set aside. Add the sage and garlic to the frying pan and cook for 1 minute. Top the bruschetta with the mushrooms and mozzarella and spoon the sage butter over to serve. Makes 6.

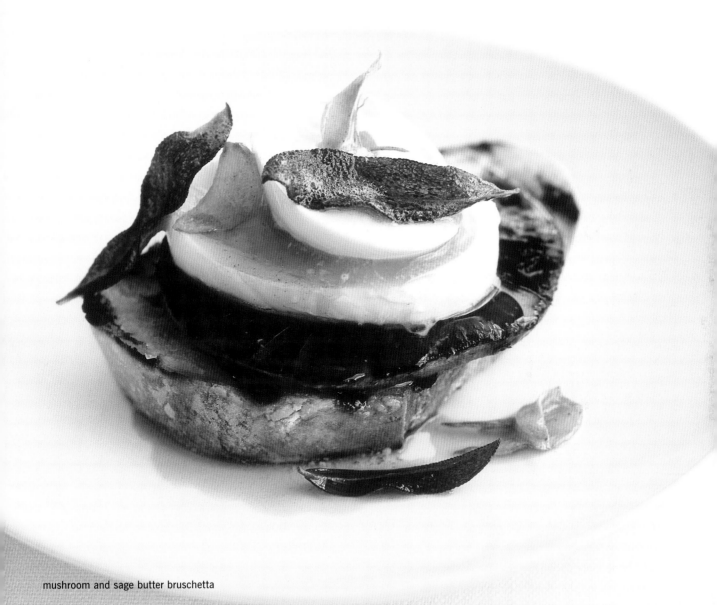

mushroom and sage butter bruschetta

salt and vinegar chunky chips

1½kg (3 lb) floury potatoes, washed, peeled and cut into chips
⅓ cup (80ml/2½ fl oz) olive oil
sea salt and cracked black pepper
¼ cup chopped green onions (scallions)
½ teaspoon brown sugar
½ cup (125ml/4 fl oz) white wine vinegar

Preheat the oven to 200°C (400°F). Place the potatoes, oil, salt and pepper in a bowl and toss to coat. Place the potatoes in a baking dish and roast for 50–55 minutes or until golden and crispy. Combine the green onions, sugar and vinegar in a jar and shake to combine. Serve the chips with the vinegar mixture on the side. Serves 4–6.

warm lemon and oregano broccolini

3 x 160g (5¾ oz) bunches broccolini, trimmed
lemon and oregano dressing
3 tablespoons olive oil
3 cloves garlic, finely sliced
1½ tablespoons lemon zest
1 tablespoon oregano leaves
1 tablespoon lemon juice
sea salt and cracked black pepper

To make the dressing, heat the oil in a small saucepan over medium heat. Add the garlic, lemon zest and oregano and cook, stirring, for 1 minute or until the garlic is soft. Add the lemon juice and cook for 1 minute, stirring, then add salt and pepper. Set aside and keep warm. Blanch the broccolini in a saucepan of boiling water for 1–2 minutes or until just tender. Drain and serve with the warm dressing. Serves 6.

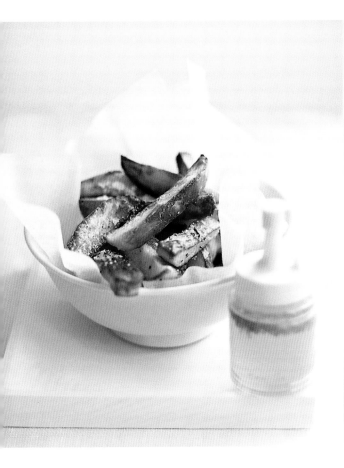

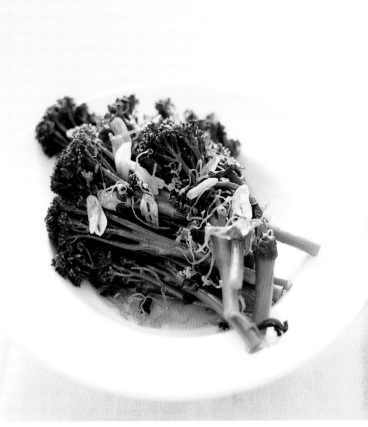

salt and vinegar chunky chips   warm lemon and oregano broccolini

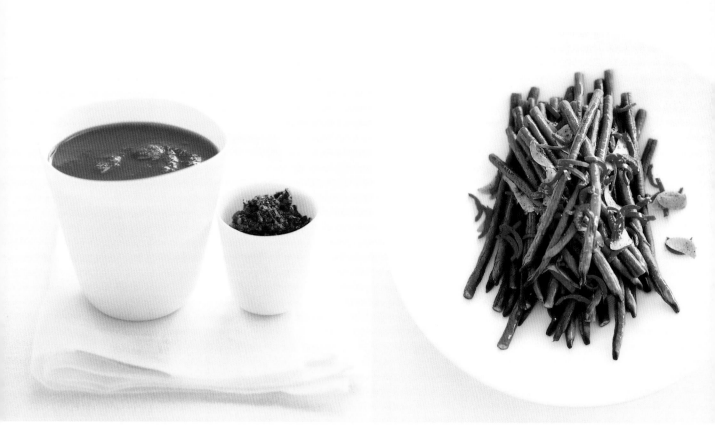

roast tomato soup   chilli salted snake beans

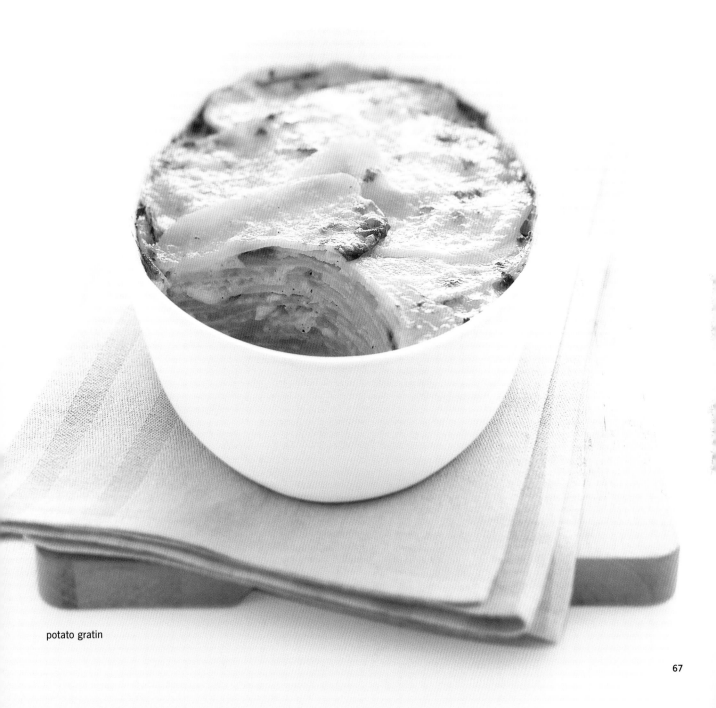

potato gratin

roast tomato soup

2kg (4 lb) vine-ripened tomatoes, halved

1 head garlic, whole and unpeeled

2 tablespoons olive oil

sea salt and cracked black pepper

3 cups (750ml/24 fl oz) chicken or vegetable stock

2–3 teaspoons sugar

1 quantity mint pesto (recipe, page 90)

Preheat the oven to 180°C (350°F). Place the tomatoes and garlic on two baking trays lined with non-stick baking paper. Drizzle with the oil and sprinkle with salt and pepper. Bake for 40 minutes or until the tomatoes are very soft. Allow to cool slightly. Squeeze the garlic flesh from its skin and process in a blender with the tomatoes and any juice from the baking trays, in 2 batches until smooth. Cook the tomato mixture, stock and sugar in a large saucepan over medium heat for 6 minutes, stirring occasionally. Ladle the soup into bowls or mugs and serve with mint pesto. Serves 4–6.

chilli salted snake beans

500g (1 lb) snake or green beans, halved

2 teaspoons sesame oil

3 long red chillies, seeded and finely sliced

2 cloves garlic, finely sliced

sea salt and cracked black pepper

Place the beans in a steamer over boiling water and cook until tender. Place the sesame oil in a hot wok with the chillies, garlic, salt and pepper. Cook for 2 minutes, then toss with the beans. Serves 6.

potato gratin

600g (1¼ lb) floury potatoes

20g (¾ oz) butter, melted

½ cup (125ml/4 fl oz) (single or pouring) cream

½ cup (125ml/4 fl oz) milk

¼ teaspoon ground nutmeg

1 brown onion, finely sliced

2 garlic cloves, crushed

sea salt and cracked black pepper

Preheat the oven to 180°C (350°F). Peel and thinly slice the potatoes. Brush a 1 litre (32 fl oz) capacity ovenproof dish with the butter. Place the cream, milk and nutmeg in a small saucepan over medium heat until just boiling and remove from the heat. Layer the potato, onion, garlic, salt and pepper in the dish finishing with a layer of potato. Pour over the warm cream mixture and bake in the oven for 45 minutes or until the potato is tender. Serves 6.

Asian greens with oyster sauce

1 teaspoon sesame oil

1 clove garlic, chopped

2 tablespoons shredded ginger

¼ cup (60ml/2 fl oz) oyster sauce

¼ cup (60ml/2 fl oz) Chinese rice wine

¼ cup (60ml/2 fl oz) salt-reduced soy sauce

2 tablespoons brown sugar

1 bunch (400g/14 oz) choy sum, trimmed

1 bunch (400g/14 oz) gai larn, trimmed

Heat the sesame oil in a small saucepan over medium heat. Add the garlic and ginger and cook for 1–2 minutes. Add the oyster sauce, rice wine, soy sauce and sugar and simmer for 5 minutes or until slightly reduced and thickened. Cut the bunches of greens in half and blanch in a saucepan of boiling water for 1–2 minutes or until just tender. Drain. To serve, place the greens on a plate and spoon over the sauce. Serves 4.

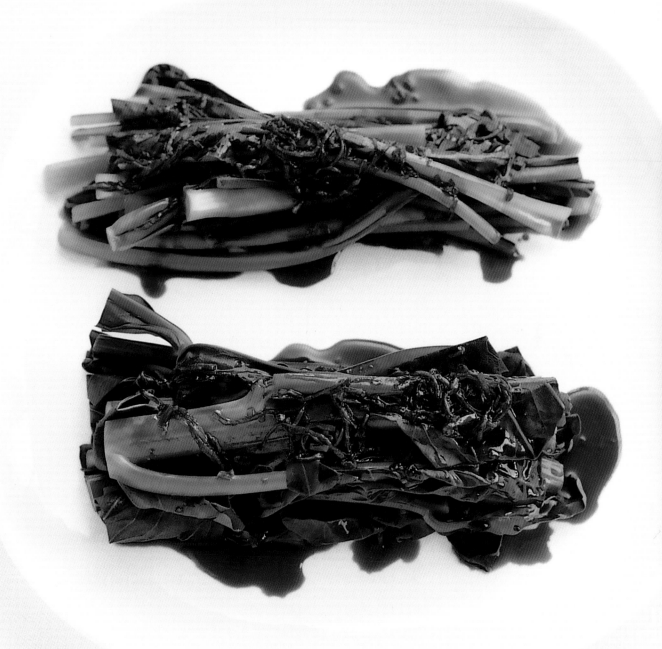

Asian greens with oyster sauce

vegetable tempura

1 eggplant (aubergine), sliced lengthways

12 spears asparagus, trimmed

500g (1 lb) Japanese pumpkin, thinly sliced

12 green beans, trimmed

peanut oil, for deep-frying

tempura batter

2 cups (300g/10½ oz) plain (all-purpose) flour

2 cups (500ml/16 fl oz) chilled soda water

soy dipping sauce

¼ cup (60ml/2 fl oz) mirin (see glossary)

2 tablespoons soy sauce

2 tablespoons water

1 teaspoon finely grated ginger

To make the dipping sauce, cook the mirin, soy sauce, water and ginger in a small saucepan over medium heat for 3–4 minutes. Set aside and keep warm.

To make the tempura batter (it is important to do this just before cooking), place the flour in a bowl and pour over the cold soda water. Stir to just combine; the batter should be quite lumpy, not smooth.

Heat the oil in a large saucepan over medium–high heat. Dip the vegetables into the batter a few at a time, coating them well. Fry the battered vegetables in batches for 2–3 minutes or until tender and very light golden. Keep warm in a low oven while cooking the remaining vegetables. Serve with the soy dipping sauce. Serves 4–6.

grilled polenta with balsamic mushrooms

4½ cups (1.25 litres/36 fl oz) chicken or vegetable stock

1 cup (180g/6 oz) instant or regular polenta

40g (1½ oz) butter

½ cup grated parmesan cheese

sea salt and cracked black pepper

vegetable oil, for brushing

balsamic mushrooms

40g (1½ oz) butter

1 clove garlic, sliced

250g (8 oz) shiitake mushrooms, thickly sliced

250g (8 oz) swiss brown mushrooms

1¾ cups (435ml/14 fl oz) beef or vegetable stock

1½ tablespoons balsamic vinegar

2 teaspoons brown sugar

1½ tablespoons chopped flat-leaf parsley leaves

Place the stock in a large saucepan over medium heat and bring to the boil. Pour in the polenta slowly in a thin stream, whisking so it doesn't form lumps. Stir for 5 minutes for instant or 20 minutes for regular polenta, or until the polenta starts to leave the side of the pan. Stir through the butter, parmesan, salt and pepper. Pour into a lightly greased 20 x 30cm (8 x 12 in) shallow tin. Refrigerate for 40 minutes or until the polenta is set.

To make the balsamic mushrooms, heat a large non-stick frying pan over medium heat. Add the butter and garlic and cook for 1 minute. Add the mushrooms and cook for 4 minutes or until golden. Add the stock, vinegar and sugar and simmer for 6 minutes or until the liquid is reduced by half. Remove the polenta from the tin and slice into 8 long triangles. Brush lightly with oil. Cook on a hot char-grill (broiler) for 4 minutes or until softened and heated through. To serve, place the polenta on plates and top with the balsamic mushrooms and chopped parsley. Serves 4.

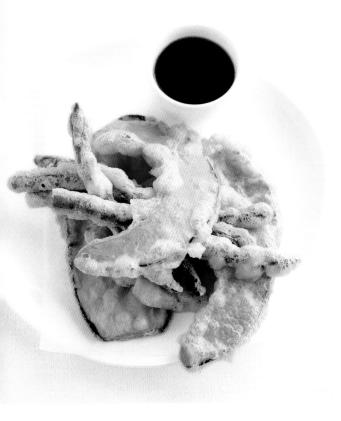

vegetable tempura

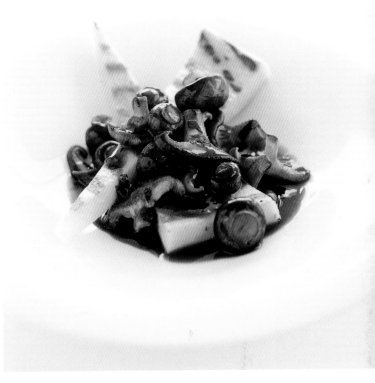

grilled polenta with balsamic mushrooms

vegetable mains

When the donna hay team was asked to nominate their absolute favourite recipes, a surprising number of the responses turned out to be vegie based. The reason they were so popular is not hard to fathom, as closer inspection reveals these dishes tick all the boxes of great taste, good health, simple preparation and hearty serves. This selection will have even dedicated carnivores lining up for seconds.

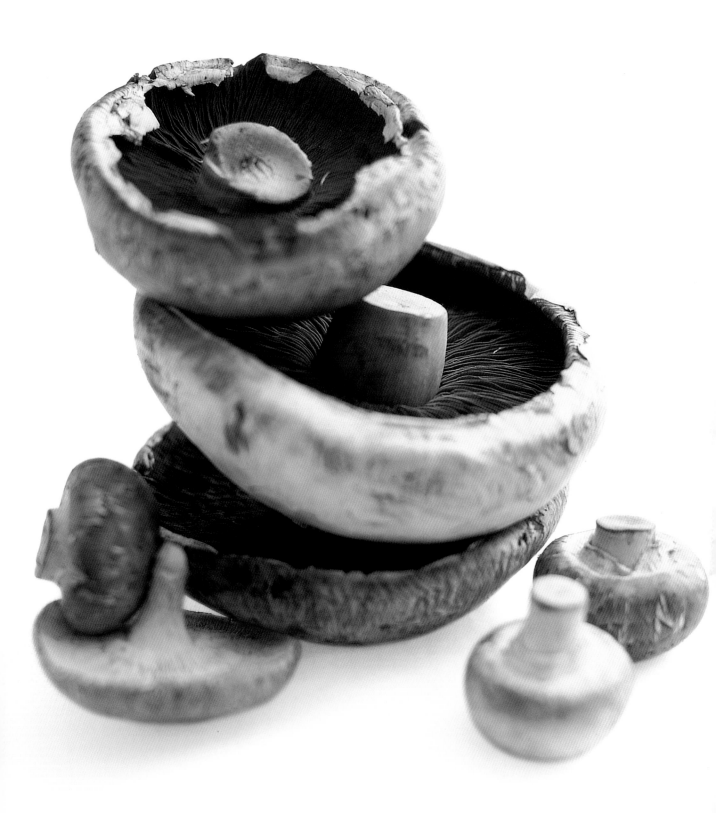

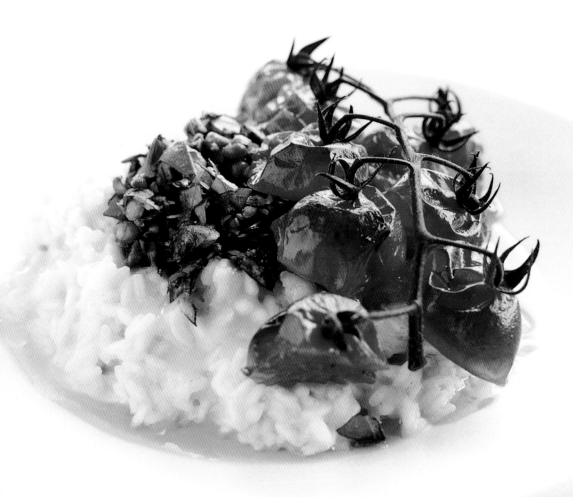

basil risotto with roast tomatoes

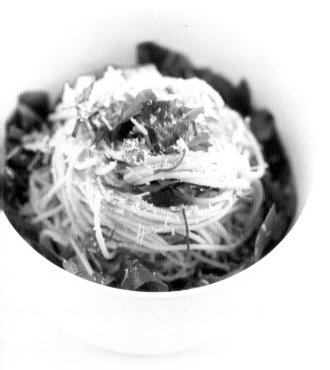

chilli, rocket and parmesan pasta

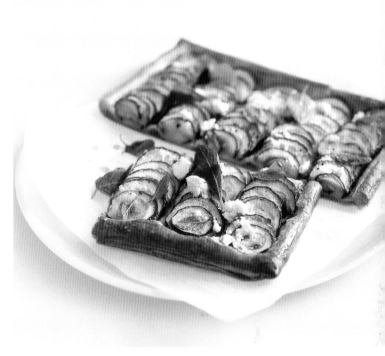

zucchini, mint and fetta tart

basil risotto with roast tomatoes

4 vines or 24 individual cherry tomatoes

olive oil, for drizzling

20g (¾ oz) butter

1 tablespoon olive oil, extra

1 onion, chopped

2 cloves garlic, sliced

5½ cups (1.4 litres/44 fl oz) chicken or vegetable stock

2 cups arborio or other risotto rice

⅓ cup finely grated parmesan cheese

1 quantity rough pesto (recipe, page 90)

Preheat the oven to 180°C (350°F). Place the tomatoes in a baking dish and drizzle with olive oil. Bake for 1 hour or until soft. To make the risotto, heat a large saucepan over medium heat. Cook the butter, extra oil, onion and garlic for 6–8 minutes. In a separate saucepan over medium heat, bring the stock to a slow simmer. Add the rice to the onion, stirring for 2 minutes or until translucent. Add the hot stock, 1 cup at a time, stirring continuously until each cup of stock is absorbed and the rice is al dente (around 25–30 minutes). Stir in the parmesan and serve in bowls topped with rough pesto, the tomatoes and drizzle with baking dish oil. Serves 4.

chilli, rocket and parmesan pasta

400g (14 oz) spaghetti

2 tablespoons olive oil

2 cloves garlic, chopped

2 long red chillies, seeded and sliced

2 teaspoons finely grated lemon rind

¼ cup (60ml/ 2 fl oz) lemon juice

1 x 100g (3½ oz) bunch rocket (arugula), roughly chopped

½ cup finely grated parmesan cheese

Cook the spaghetti in a large saucepan of salted and rapidly boiling water for 10–12 minutes or until al dente. Drain. Heat the oil in a large non-stick frying pan over medium heat. Add the garlic, chillies and lemon rind and cook for 1–2 minutes or until light golden. Toss with the lemon juice, rocket, pasta and half of the parmesan. Serve with remaining parmesan. Serves 4.

zucchini, mint and fetta tart

1 x 200g (7 oz) sheet store-bought butter puff pastry, thawed

4 zucchini (courgettes), thinly sliced

1 tablespoon finely grated lemon rind

1 tablespoon olive oil

sea salt and cracked black pepper

1 egg, lightly beaten

150g (5¼ oz) fetta cheese, crumbled

½ cup mint leaves

olive oil, extra, to serve

Preheat the oven to 200°C (400°F). Place the pastry on a baking tray lined with non-stick baking paper. Score a 1cm (½ in) border around the edge of the pastry with a sharp knife. Place the zucchini, lemon rind, oil, salt and pepper in a medium bowl and toss to coat. Layer the zucchini mixture on the pastry and brush the edges with egg. Bake for 20–25 minutes or until the pastry is puffed and golden and the zucchini is cooked. Top with the fetta, mint and extra oil. Serves 4.

vegetable stir-fry

1 tablespoon peanut oil

2 long red chillies, seeded and sliced

2 onions, sliced into thin wedges

½ teaspoon Chinese five-spice powder

2 cloves garlic, sliced

200g (7 oz) green beans, trimmed

1 red capsicum (bell pepper), sliced

2 zucchini (courgettes), sliced

2 cups broccoli florets

200g (7 oz) snow peas (mange tout), trimmed

2 tablespoons oyster sauce

2 tablespoons small basil leaves

¼ cup roasted unsalted cashews

Heat a wok or large non-stick frying pan over high heat. Cook the oil, chillies, onions, five-spice and garlic for 2 minutes. Add the beans, capsicum, zucchini, broccoli and snow peas and stir-fry for 4–5 minutes or until tender. Toss through the oyster sauce. Sprinkle with the basil and cashews. Serves 4.

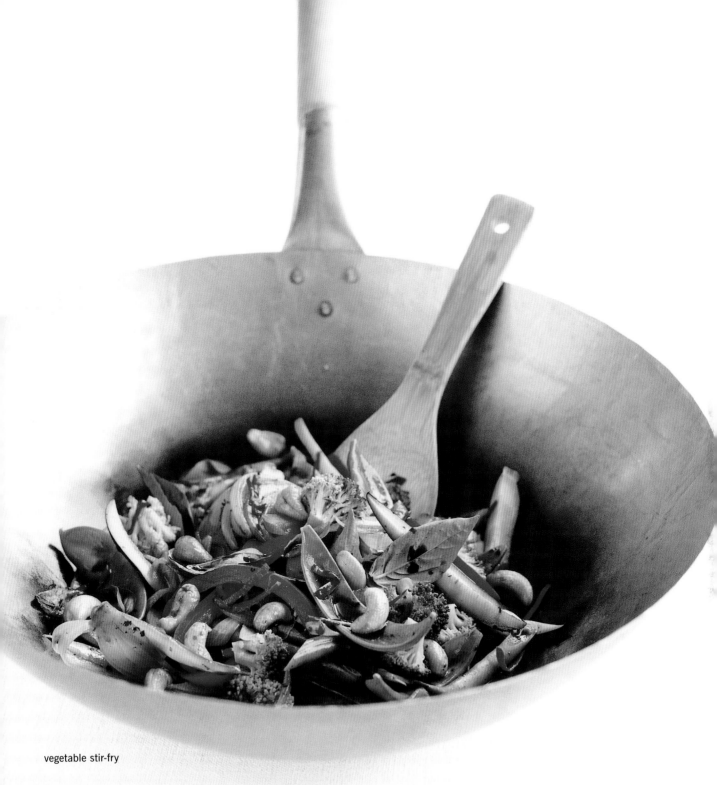
vegetable stir-fry

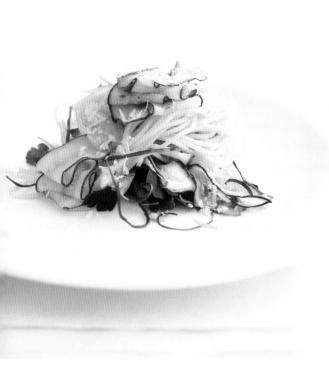

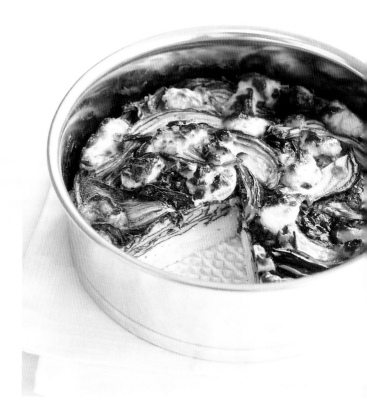

pan-fried zucchini and chilli pasta

goat's cheese, polenta and spinach bake

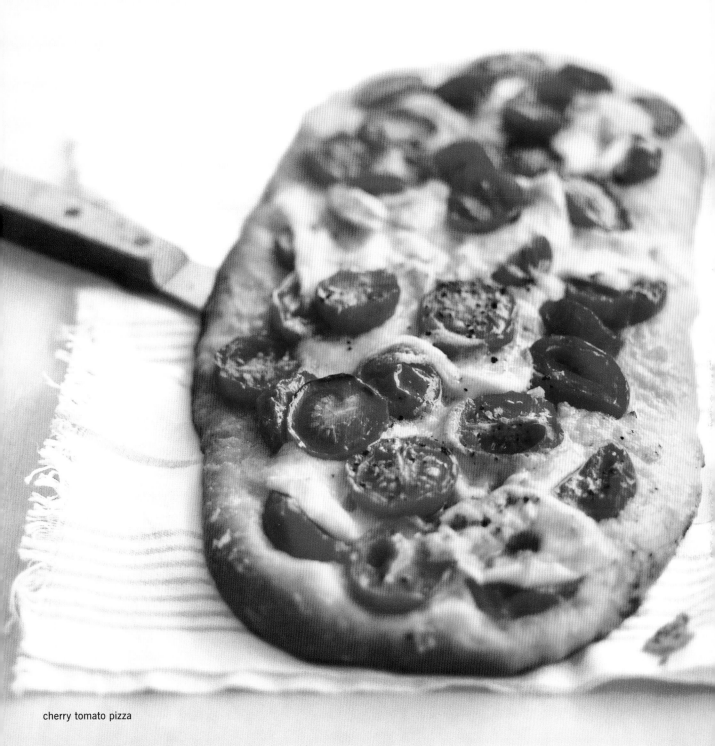

cherry tomato pizza

pan-fried zucchini and chilli pasta

400g (14 oz) spaghetti

2 tablespoons olive oil

2 cloves garlic, thinly sliced

4 zucchini, thinly sliced lengthways

1 long red chilli, seeded and thinly sliced lengthways

1 tablespoon finely grated lemon rind

2 tablespoons lemon juice

sea salt and cracked black pepper

1 cup flat-leaf parsley leaves

¼ cup finely grated parmesan cheese

Cook the pasta in a large saucepan of salted boiling water until al dente. Drain, set aside and keep warm.

Heat a medium non-stick frying pan over high heat. Add the oil and garlic and cook for 1 minute, add the zucchini and chilli and cook for a further 2–3 minutes or until zucchini is tender. Stir through the lemon rind and lemon juice. Add to the pasta, salt, pepper, parsley and parmesan and toss to combine. Serves 4.

goat's cheese, polenta and spinach bake

1 quantity soft polenta (recipe, page 90)

150g (5¼ oz) English spinach, trimmed and washed

1 x 100g (3½ oz) red onion, sliced

6 eggs, lightly beaten

½ cup (125ml/4 fl oz) (single or pouring) cream

80g (2¾ oz) goat's cheese, crumbled

Preheat the oven to 180°C (350°F). Lightly grease a 20cm (8 in) springform tin and line the base with non-stick baking paper. Spread the polenta over the base of the tin, top with the spinach and red onion. Whisk together the eggs and cream, pour over the spinach and onion and top with the goat's cheese. Place tin on a baking tray and cook for 40 minutes or until set. Serves 4.

cherry tomato pizza

1 quantity pizza base (recipe, page 90)

olive oil, for brushing

sea salt

2 x 250g (8 oz) punnets cherry tomatoes, halved

200g (7 oz) fresh mozzarella cheese, sliced

cracked black pepper

Preheat the oven to 200°C (400°F). Divide the dough in 2 and roll out to 1cm (½ in) thickness, brush with the oil and sprinkle with the salt. Top each base with the tomatoes and mozzarella and sprinkle with the pepper. Cook for 20 minutes or until the tops are golden and the bases crispy. Makes 2.

spinach and ricotta cannelloni

1 quantity basic tomato sauce (recipe, page 88)

   or 500 ml (16 fl oz) store-bought tomato pasta sauce

4 large fresh lasagne sheets, halved lengthways

½ cup finely grated parmesan cheese

spinach ricotta filling

2 x 500g (1 lb) bunches English spinach, trimmed

750g (1½ lb) fresh ricotta

1 cup finely grated parmesan cheese

2 tablespoons chopped flat-leaf parsley leaves

1 tablespoon chopped dill

½ cup fresh breadcrumbs

sea salt and cracked black pepper

Preheat the oven to 180°C (350°F). To make the filling, blanch the spinach in a saucepan of boiling water for 5 seconds, then drain, squeeze out any excess moisture, and chop. Combine the spinach, ricotta, parmesan, parsley, dill, breadcrumbs, salt and pepper. Spread one-third of the basic tomato sauce over the base of a lightly greased 20 x 30cm (8 x 12 in) ovenproof dish. Lay a lasagne sheet on a flat surface, spoon on some ricotta filling and roll up. Place in the baking dish, seam-side down. Repeat with the remaining filling and sheets. Pour the remaining tomato sauce over the cannelloni and bake for 25–30 minutes or until the top is browned and the cannelloni are heated through. To serve, sprinkle with parmesan. Serves 4.

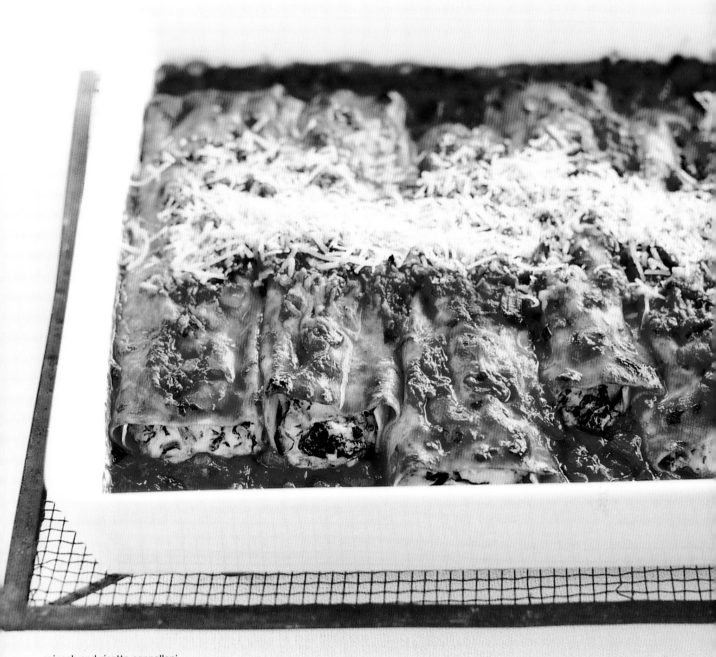

spinach and ricotta cannelloni

free-form ratatouille tart

1 quantity shortcrust pastry (recipe, page 90)
ratatouille filling
1 head garlic, unpeeled, cut in half horizontally
2 brown onions, peeled and quartered
2 red capsicums (bell peppers), seeded and quartered
2 x 230g (7⅞ oz) eggplants (aubergines), cut into wedges
4 roma tomatoes, halved
3 zucchini (courgettes), quartered
2 tablespoons olive oil
sea salt and cracked black pepper
200g (7 oz) fetta, roughly crumbled
1 tablespoon marjoram leaves

Preheat the oven to 180°C (350°F). To make the filling, place the garlic, onions, capsicums, eggplants, tomatoes and zucchini on a large baking tray, drizzle with the oil and sprinkle with salt and pepper. Bake for 1 hour or until the vegetables are golden and slightly dried. Allow to cool then squeeze the flesh from the garlic skins and set aside.

Roll out the pastry on a lightly floured surface into a roughly 30cm (12 in) round that is 3mm (⅛ in) thick. Place on a baking tray, spread with the garlic and top with the vegetables, fetta and marjoram, leaving a 6cm (2½ in) border. Fold over the edges of the pastry to make a raised edge. Chill for 20 minutes. Bake for 45 minutes or until the pastry is golden and crisp. Serve warm or cold. Serves 6.

+ This type of free-form tart works well with any filling combination – including vegetables with meat or chicken – as long as the ingredients are firm. The cooked tart needs to be solid enough to be sliced for serving. When making it on a hot day, you may need to chill the tart for a longer time before cooking it.

roast vegetable frittata

600g (20 oz) orange sweet potato (kumara) or pumpkin,
    peeled and chopped
1 red capsicum (bell pepper), cut into 8 pieces
2 zucchini (courgettes), quartered
4 baby/chat (new) potatoes, quartered
olive oil and sea salt for sprinkling
frittata mix
6 eggs
1 cup (250ml/8 fl oz) (single or pouring) cream
½ cup grated aged cheddar or parmesan cheese
2 tablespoons shredded basil leaves
cracked black pepper
toast, to serve

Preheat the oven to 180°C (350°F). Place the sweet potato or pumpkin, capsicum, zucchini and potatoes on a baking tray lined with non-stick baking paper. Drizzle with oil and sprinkle with salt. Bake for 40 minutes or until soft and golden. Place the roast vegetables in a 20cm (8 in) non-stick frying pan.

To make the frittata, whisk together the eggs, cream, cheese, basil and pepper. Pour over the vegetables in the frying pan and cook over low heat for 8–10 minutes or until the frittata begins to set. Place the frittata under a preheated hot grill (broiler) and cook for 2 minutes or until golden. Allow to stand for 5 minutes before slicing into thick wedges. Serve immediately, with toast if desired. Serves 4–6.

+ Other combinations of cooked vegetables can be used to make frittata – char-grilled eggplant (aubergine) and mushrooms work really well. You can also use leftover roast vegetables and add ingredients such as chopped cooked chicken, drained canned tuna, other kinds of hard cheeses and fresh herbs.

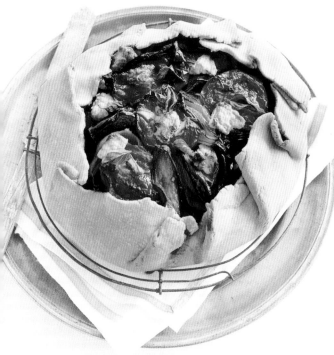

free-form ratatouille tart

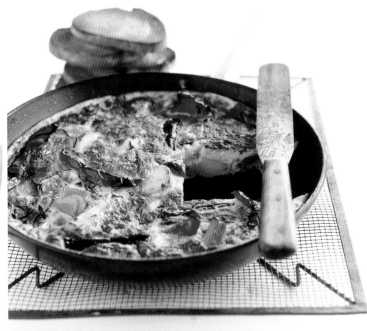

roast vegetable frittata

vegetable lasagne

8 vine-ripened tomatoes, thickly sliced

3 orange sweet potatoes (kumara), peeled and thinly sliced

2 eggplants (aubergines), thickly sliced

3 red capsicums (bell peppers), cut into 8 pieces

5 zucchini (courgettes), thickly sliced lengthways

4 field mushrooms, sliced

sea salt

375g (13¼ oz) fresh lasagne sheets+

ricotta filling

1kg (2 lb) fresh ricotta cheese

¼ cup chopped basil leaves

¼ cup chopped flat-leaf parsley leaves

2 eggs

¾ cup (185ml/6 fl oz) (single or pouring) cream

sea salt and cracked black pepper

1 cup grated mozzarella cheese

Preheat the oven to 180°C (350°F). Place the tomatoes, sweet potatoes, eggplants, capsicums, zucchini and mushrooms on baking trays lined with non-stick baking paper. Sprinkle with salt and bake for 40 minutes or until tender and golden.

To make the ricotta filling, combine the ricotta, basil, parsley, eggs, cream, salt and pepper. Grease a 32 x 22cm (12¾ x 8½ in) or similar ovenproof baking dish. Line with some of the lasagne sheets. Place half of the vegetables on top, then another lasagne sheet. Spoon over half of the ricotta mixture, then place another layer of lasagne sheets on top. Continue layering, finishing with the ricotta mixture. Sprinkle with the mozzarella and bake for 45 minutes or until the vegetables are soft. Serves 6–8.

+ You can also use dried lasagne sheets that have been cooked in boiling water until soft.

pea and zucchini risotto

6 cups (1.5 litres/48 fl oz) chicken or vegetable stock

½ cup (125ml/4 fl oz) white wine

40g (1½ oz) butter

2 leeks, trimmed and sliced

2 cloves garlic, crushed

2 cups arborio rice

2 teaspoons olive oil

3 zucchini (courgettes), sliced

1½ cups frozen peas

65g (2¼ oz) baby spinach leaves

¼ cup chopped flat-leaf parsley leaves

sea salt and cracked black pepper

shaved parmesan cheese, to serve

lemon wedges, to serve

Place the stock and wine in a large saucepan over medium heat. Cover and bring to a slow simmer. Melt the butter in a separate large saucepan over medium heat. Add the leeks and cook for 5 minutes or until soft. Add the garlic and rice and cook, stirring, for 2 minutes or until the rice is translucent. Pour in the hot stock, 1 cup at a time, stirring constantly, until each cup of stock is absorbed and the rice is just al dente (around 25 minutes). Heat the oil in a medium non-stick frying pan over high heat. Add the zucchini and cook for 5 minutes or until tender. Add the zucchini to the risotto, along with the peas, spinach, parsley, salt and pepper. Cook for 4 minutes or until the spinach is wilted and the peas are heated through. To serve, top with the parmesan and add lemon wedges, if desired. Serves 4.

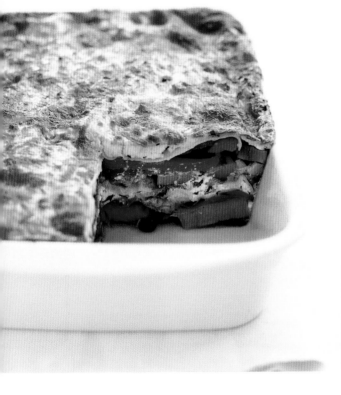

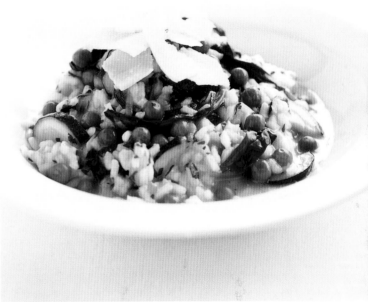

vegetable lasagne

pea and zucchini risotto

glossary, index

+ conversions

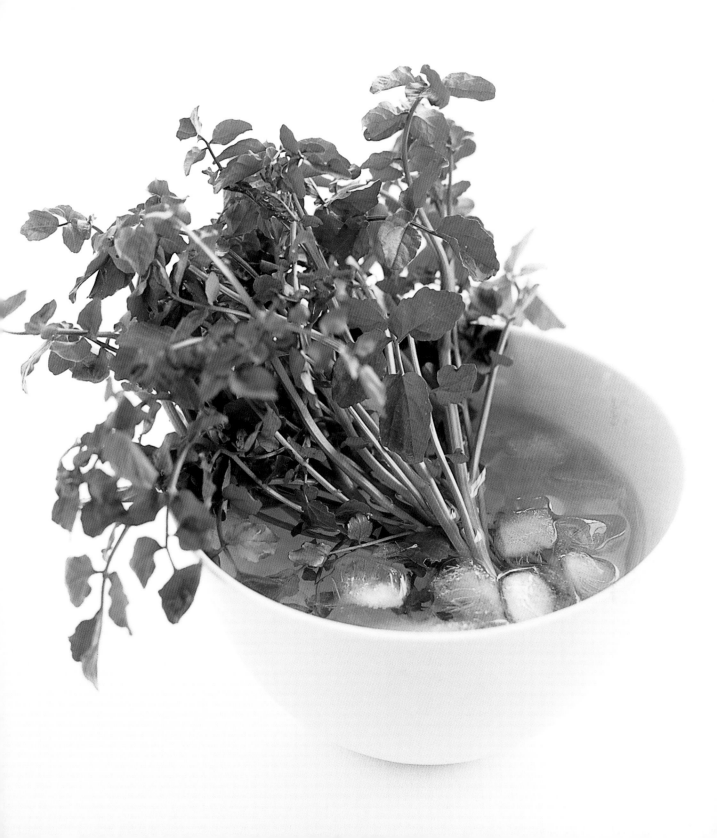

balsamic vinegar

A rich, dark colour and a sweet, mellow, almost caramel flavour distinguish balsamic from other wine vinegars. Made from trebbiano grapes in Modena, Italy, it is aged for 5 to 30 years, or more. The older the balsamic, the better (and more expensive) and the less you'll need to use. Cheaper ones may need to be balanced with some sugar. It should not be used as a substitute for regular vinegar.

roasted tomato sauce

1kg (2 lb) ripe roma tomatoes
5 cloves garlic
2 tablespoons extra virgin olive oil
1 teaspoon red wine vinegar
1 teaspoon caster (superfine) sugar
sea salt and cracked black pepper
1 cup basil leaves

Preheat the oven to 200°C (400°F). Cut a shallow 2cm (¾ in) cross into the base of each tomato. Place the tomatoes and garlic in a baking dish lined with non-stick baking paper. Roast for 15–20 minutes or until the skin starts to peel away and the tomatoes are tender. Remove from the oven and allow to cool slightly. Peel the tomatoes and the garlic and roughly chop. Place them in a bowl, add the oil, vinegar, sugar, salt, pepper and basil and stir well to combine. Makes 2¾ cups.

buttermilk

Originally the name given to the slightly tangy liquid left over when cream is separated from milk, these days buttermilk is manufactured by adding cultures to low- or no-fat milk. Contrary to what the name may suggest, buttermilk is a low-fat ingredient. Use in sauces, marinades, dressings and baking.

buttermilk (ranch) dressing

3 tablespoons buttermilk
¼ cup (60g/2 fl oz) sour cream
2 teaspoons white wine vinegar
1 teaspoon Dijon mustard
2 teaspoons chopped chives
1½ teaspoons finely chopped
    flat-leaf parsley leaves

Combine the buttermilk, sour cream, vinegar and mustard in a small bowl or jar. Stir in the chives and parsley. Or stir in 75g (2⅔ oz) crumbled blue cheese for a tangy blue cheese dressing. Makes ⅔ cup.

caesar salad dressing

1 egg yolk
2 teaspoons Dijon mustard
1 clove garlic, chopped
2 tablespoons lemon juice
3 anchovy fillets
¼ cup finely grated parmesan cheese
½ cup (125ml/4 fl oz) vegetable oil

Process the egg yolk, mustard, garlic, lemon juice, anchovies and parmesan in a food processor until combined. With the motor running, gradually add the oil and process until smooth. Makes ⅔ cup.

basic tomato sauce

2 teaspoons olive oil
2 cloves garlic, finely chopped
1 brown onion, finely chopped
2 x 400g (14 oz) cans crushed tomatoes
3 teaspoons sugar
¼ cup chopped basil leaves

Heat a large saucepan over medium heat. Add the oil, garlic and onion and cook for 4–5 minutes or until the onion is tender. Add the tomatoes, sugar and basil, reduce heat and simmer for 10–12 minutes or until the sauce is thick. Makes 2 cups.

capers

Capers are the small, deep green flower buds of the caper bush. Available packed either in brine or salt. Use salt-packed capers when possible, as the texture is firmer and the flavour superior. Before use, rinse thoroughly, drain and pat dry.

cheese

blue cheese

The distinctive veins and flavour of blue cheeses are achieved by adding a cultured mould. Most have a crumbly texture and acidic taste, which becomes rounded and more mellow with age. Blue cheeses are best served at room temperature.

bocconcini

Fresh Italian mozzarella balls, available in a variety of sizes, usually made from cow's milk. Sold in water or a brine solution in delicatessens and supermarkets.

fetta

Made from goat's, sheep's or cow's milk, fetta is a salty, crumbly cheese which is often stored in brine to extend its shelf life.

goat's cheese

Goat's milk has a characteristic tart flavour, so cheese made from it, sometimes labelled chèvre, has a sharp, slightly acidic taste. Young goat's cheese is milder and creamier than mature cheese.

haloumi

Firm white Cypriot cheese made from sheep's milk. It has a stringy texture and is usually sold in brine. Available from delicatessens and some supermarkets. Holds its shape during grilling and frying, so is ideal for kebabs.

mozzarella

Italian in origin, mozzarella is the mild cheese of pizza, lasagne and tomato salads. It's made by cutting and spinning (or stringing) the curd to achieve a smooth, elastic consistency.

buffalo mozzarella

Made from water buffalo's milk, this is considered to be the best mozzarella. It is sold in whey at specialty food stores.

parmesan

Italy's favourite hard, granular cheese is made from cow's milk. Parmigiano reggiano is the Rolls Royce variety, made under strict guidelines in the Emilia-Romagna region and aged for an average of 2 years. Grana padano mainly comes from Lombardy. It's aged for 15 months.

ricotta

A creamy, finely grained white cheese. Ricotta means "recooked" in Italian, a reference to the way the cheese is produced by heating the whey left over from making other cheese varieties.

Chinese five-spice powder

This combination of cinnamon, Sichuan pepper, star anise, clove and fennel is available from Asian food stores and most supermarkets.

Chinese rice wine

Similar to dry sherry, Chinese cooking wine is a blend of glutinous rice, millet, a special yeast and the local spring waters of Shao Hsing, where it is made, in northern China. It is sold in Asian supermarkets, often labelled "shao hsing".

Dijon mustard

Originating from the French city of the same name, Dijon mustard is pale yellow in colour and ranges from mild to very hot. It is made from husked black mustard seeds blended with wine, salt and spices.

fish sauce

An amber-coloured liquid drained from salted, fermented fish and used to add flavour to Thai and Vietnamese dishes. Available from supermarkets and Asian food stores, this pungent sauce is often labelled "nam pla".

hoisin sauce

A thick, sweet Chinese sauce made from fermented soybeans, sugar, salt and red rice. Used as a dipping sauce or marinade and as the sauce for Peking duck. Hoisin is available from Asian food stores and most supermarkets.

kaffir lime leaves

Fragrant leaves with a distinctive double leaf structure, used crushed or shredded in Thai dishes. Available fresh or dried from Asian food stores and greengrocers.

lentils

An excellent source of protein lending colour, texture and earthy flavour to soups, salads and braises. Colours range from green and brown to split, or dehusked, red.

mirin

Extremely sweet low-alcohol wine made from glutinous rice. Mirin is used in Japanese dishes and is an essential ingredient in teriyaki sauce. Available from Asian food stores and most supermarkets. Use sweet white wine if it's not available.

olives

Black olives are more mature and less salty than the green variety. Choose firm olives with good colour and a fruity taste.

Ligurian/wild olives

Sold as Ligurian olives, wild olives are uncultivated and grow close to the ground in clusters. This small variety of olive can range in colour from pale mustard to dark purple and black. The limited flesh has a nutty flavour that makes them a great substitute for peanuts. Niçoise olives are similar in size and flavour.

Kalamata olives

Of Greek origin, the large Kalamata olives have an intense flavour, which makes them the ideal choice for Greek salads. They are sometimes sold cracked or split to better absorb the flavour of the oil or vinegar in which they are stored.

olive oil

Olive oil is graded according to its flavour, aroma and acidity. Extra virgin is the highest-quality oil; it contains no more than 1 per cent acid. Virgin is the next best; it contains 1.5 per cent or less acid and may have a slightly fruitier taste than extra virgin. Bottles labelled "olive oil" contain a combination of refined and unrefined virgin olive oil. Light olive oil is the least pure in quality and intensity of flavour; it is not lower in fat. Colours vary from deep green through to gold and very light yellow.

pancetta

A cured and rolled Italian-style meat that is like prosciutto but less salty and with a softer texture. It can be eaten uncooked.

pastry

Make your own or use one of the many store-bought varieties.

puff pastry

This pastry is time-consuming and quite difficult to make, so many cooks opt to use store-bought puff pastry. It can be bought in blocks from patisseries or bought in both block and sheet forms from the supermarket. You may need to layer several sheets together to achieve the desired thickness.

shortcrust pastry

A savoury or sweet pastry that is available ready-made in blocks and frozen sheets. Keep a supply for last-minute pies and desserts, or make your own.

shortcrust pastry recipe

2 cups (300g/10½ oz) plain
   (all-purpose) flour
180g (6¼ oz) butter
2–3 tablespoons iced water

Process the flour and butter in a food processor until the mixture resembles fine breadcrumbs. While the motor is running, add enough iced water to form a smooth dough. Knead very lightly then wrap the dough in plastic wrap and refrigerate for 30 minutes. When ready to use, roll out on a lightly floured surface to 3mm (⅛ in) thick. This recipe makes 350g (12 oz), which is enough to line a 25cm (10 in) pie dish or tart tin.

pesto

From an Italian word meaning "to crush or pound", pesto has evolved from the basil original to include a range of pastes based on herbs, cheese, oil and nuts.

mint pesto recipe

1 cup mint leaves
½ cup flat-leaf parsley leaves
¼ cup roasted pine nuts
¼ cup finely grated parmesan cheese
¼ cup (60ml/2 fl oz) olive oil

Roughly chop the mint, parsley, pine nuts and parmesan cheese in a blender or food processor. Add the olive oil and blend until combined and slightly thickened.

rough pesto recipe

1 cup basil leaves, roughly chopped
1 clove garlic, crushed
⅓ cup finely grated parmesan cheese
¼ cup roasted pine nuts, roughly chopped
⅓ cup (60ml/2 fl oz) olive oil

Combine the basil, garlic, parmesan, pine nuts and oil in a small bowl or jar.

pizza base

1 teaspoon yeast
¼ teaspoon sugar
¾ cup (185ml/6 fl oz) lukewarm water
1¼ cups (190g/6¾ oz) plain
   (all-purpose) flour
½ teaspoon salt

Place the yeast, sugar and water in a bowl and mix to combine. Set aside in a warm place for 10 minutes or until bubbles appear. Place the flour and salt in a bowl. Add the yeast mixture and stir until it starts to come together, then use your hands to mix until a dough forms. Set aside in a warm place for 20 minutes or until the dough has doubled in size.

prosciutto

Italian ham that has been salted and air-dried for up to 2 years. The paper-thin slices are eaten raw or used to flavour cooked dishes.

polenta

A fine, dry cornmeal that, when cooked with water, milk and butter, forms a thick, creamy paste. Use the instant or quick-cook variety for speed and convenience. You can serve polenta wherever you would have mashed potato. Or allow it to set in a shallow cake tin, cut into small pieces and grill until golden.

risoni

A small, rice-shaped pasta used in soups and salads and to thicken and accompany stews. Greek orzo is very similar in size and can be substituted.

soft polenta

1 cup (250ml/8 fl oz) hot water
1 cup (250ml/8 fl oz) milk
½ cup polenta
30g (1 oz) butter
½ cup finely grated parmesan cheese
sea salt and cracked black pepper

Place the water and milk in a small saucepan over medium heat and bring to the boil. Gradually pour in the polenta, whisking until smooth. Reduce the heat to low and stir with a wooden spoon for 5 minutes or until the polenta starts to leave the side of the pan. Stir through the butter, parmesan, salt and pepper.

soy sauce

Soy sauce is made from fermented soybeans, salt and water. The Japanese variety is often more refined than the Chinese. Darker soys are generally older than the fresher, light varieties and may have molasses added for a richer, sweeter flavour. Salt-reduced versions are also now available from most supermarkets and Asian food stores.

Thai dressing

1 teaspoon soy sauce

2 tablespoons fish sauce

2 tablespoons lime juice

2 tablespoons brown or palm sugar

Combine the soy sauce, fish sauce, lime juice and sugar in a jar or small bowl.

wasabi

A pungent traditional Japanese condiment made from horseradish. Available from Asian food stores.

white wine vinegar

The oldest vinegar-making process began in Orleans in France. Wine was stored in partially full oak barrels, loosely sealed and allowed to develop an acidic flavour naturally. Today that process is hastened by added cultures. The best flavour is from vinegars made from quality wines.

white wine vinegar dressing recipe

1 tablespoon olive oil

1 tablespoon white wine vinegar

Combine the oil and vinegar in a small jar or non-metallic bowl.

white beans

These small, kidney-shaped beans are often called cannellini beans. Available from delicatessens and supermarkets, either canned or dried. Dried beans need to be soaked overnight before cooking.

conversion chart

1 teaspoon = 5ml

1 Australian tablespoon = 20ml (4 teaspoons)

1 UK tablespoon = 15ml (3 teaspoons/½ fl oz)

1 cup = 250ml (8 fl oz)

liquid conversions

metric	imperial	cups
30ml	1 fl oz	⅛ cup
60ml	2 fl oz	¼ cup
80ml	2½ fl oz	⅓ cup
125ml	4 fl oz	½ cup
185ml	6 fl oz	¾ cup
250ml	8 fl oz	1 cup
375ml	12 fl oz	1½ cups
500ml	16 fl oz	2 cups
600ml	20 fl oz	2½ cups
750ml	24 fl oz	3 cups
1 litre	32 fl oz	4 cups

cup measures

1 cup sugar, white	220g	7¾ oz
1 cup plain (all-purpose) flour	150g	5¼ oz
1 cup arborio rice, uncooked	220g	7¾ oz
1 cup couscous, uncooked	180g	6¼ oz
1 cup basil leaves	45g	1⅔ oz
1 cup coriander (cilantro) leaves	40g	1½ oz
1 cup mint leaves	35g	1¼ oz
1 cup flat-leaf parsley leaves	40g	1½ oz
1 cup olives	175g	6 oz
1 cup parmesan cheese, finely grated	100g	3½ oz
1 cup green peas, frozen	170g	5⅞ oz

A new series of clever and simple recipes
from Australia's no. 1 cookbook author.

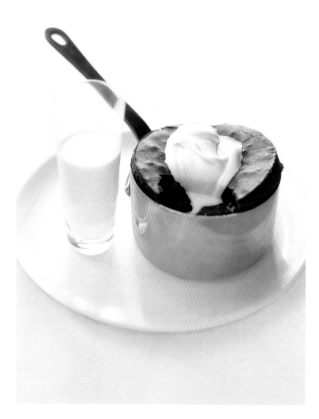

molten chocolate puddings

150g (5¼ oz) dark chocolate
100g (3½ oz) unsalted butter
2 eggs
2 egg yolks
¼ cup (55g/1⅞ oz) caster (superfine) sugar
2 tablespoons plain (all-purpose) flour, sifted
thick (double) cream to serve

Preheat the oven to 180°C (350°F). Place the chocolate and butter
in a saucepan over low heat and stir until the chocolate is melted and
smooth. Place the eggs, yolks and sugar in a bowl and whisk until
pale. Gently fold in the flour and chocolate mixture and spoon into
4 lightly greased 1 cup (250ml/8 fl oz) capacity ovenproof dishes.
Bake for 12–15 minutes or until the puddings are puffed. Top with the
cream to serve. Serves 4.

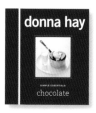

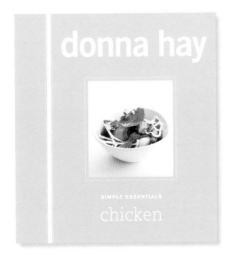

donna hay

SIMPLE ESSENTIALS
chicken

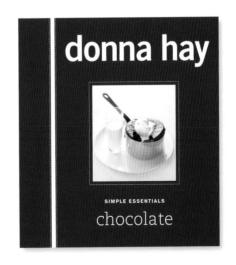

donna hay

SIMPLE ESSENTIALS
chocolate

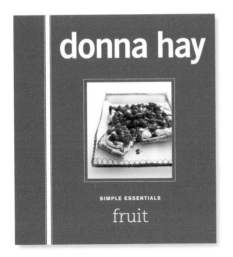

donna hay

SIMPLE ESSENTIALS
fruit

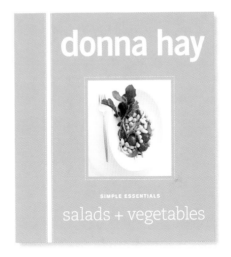

donna hay

SIMPLE ESSENTIALS
salads + vegetables

donna hay

SIMPLE ESSENTIALS

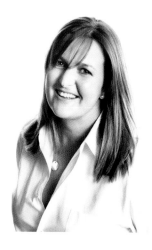

At the age of eight, Donna Hay put on an apron and never looked back. She completed formal training in home economics at technical college then moved to the world of magazine test kitchens and publishing where she established her trademark style of simple, smart and seasonal recipes all beautifully put together and photographed. It is food for every cook, every food lover, every day and every occasion. Her unique style turned her into an international food publishing phenomenon as a bestselling author, publisher of *donna hay magazine*, newspaper columnist, and creator of a homewares and food range.

books by Donna Hay: *off the shelf, modern classics book 1, modern classics book 2, the instant cook, instant entertaining, simple essentials: chicken,* and *simple essentials: chocolate,* plus more.